Yc

(and

ISBN: 1507676948
ISBN-13: 978-1507676943

For my son, who came into our world and turned it upside down.

"Our mothers always remain the strangest, craziest people we've ever met."

— Marguerite Duras

CONCEPTION IS NOT IMMACULATE

September 26

Tom and I made the momentous decision to try for a baby three months ago, immediately after getting hitched in June. "It might take us ages," I'd told him "and we're not getting any younger – well, you aren't anyway" (I'm 30 and he's 40).

We both have friends who have undergone long and arduous courses of fertility treatment and thought it was best to get cracking, just in case. Despite this, I've been more than a little disappointed by the persistent arrival of my period after three months of honeymoon hanky panky. Doing it when the mood takes you, it appears, is not enough. So, I've decided it's time to focus my attention and start getting scientific on this baby-making malarkey – and keep a diary about my efforts.

The first thing I've realised is how very little I really know about the female reproductive system. I understood that the menstrual cycle involved preparation for ovulation, ovulation and then the delightful monthly clear out of the womb, but I'd always been under the impression that one could conceive at any time of the month.

This was the message that was drilled into us as girls via school sex education and teen magazines. There would always be a letter on the problem page enquiring whether it was possible to get pregnant standing up/on your period/just before your period/in a swimming pool etc. and the answer was always an unequivocal YES!

However, after doing some research on exactly what goes on 'down there' I was shocked to learn that the egg, once it is released, only lives for 12 hours. Unless it meets sperm within that miniscule window, there's no chance of conceiving for another month. Even if the egg is lucky enough to meet a sperm, it must then succeed in the evidentially difficult task of embedding itself in the womb.

One wonders how anyone manages to get pregnant at that rate, but somehow that underage couple who only have sex 'just that one time' often seem to hit the bullseye. They may deem themselves unlucky but beating those odds is surely akin to winning the lottery (or at least a substantial prize on a scratch card).

Just how long will it take for me to get lucky is what I want to know?

September 28

Just how often is often enough to have sex when you're trying to conceive? According to the NHS, it's every two to three days, which seems reasonable, but according to my friend Anna that's not nearly often enough. Anna has four children – so has some level of expertise – although she freely admits they were all unplanned. Lest you get the wrong impression, she's only been careless on three occasions, not four; her two youngest are are twins.

This was in fact a double delight for her because she just loves babies and to that end is very, very eager for me to produce a sproglet for her to 'steal'.

"I'm putting you on a regime," she informed me. "I want you doing it every day or every 12-hours if you can manage it."

I told her I most certainly could not and that I had been concentrating the sexual activity around the time of ovulation (around the 14th day of my cycle). This was apparently another schoolgirl error, as ovulation might not necessarily take place when you think it will.

I couldn't even take comfort in the fact that Tom already has a daughter - Rosie - as it was 12 years since his sperm had proved itself and it could now be 'past its best', she informed me.

"You just need to keep doing it all the time," she said. "And pop your bum on a pillow to help the sperm go in," she added thoughtfully.

It's easy for her to dish out this punishing sexual schedule when she only has to look at a willy to get pregnant. I've got to be honest, despite only being married a short time, having sex every day sounds like pretty hard work, particularly as my job as a journalist often keeps me out late into the evening. However, I know she has a point and if you really want something you've got to be prepared to work for it. So, if you'll excuse me, Tom and I will be back in ten minutes…

September 29

Sex is great, most of the time, but it's much more fun when you *want* to do it rather than when you *have* to. However, the fertile window around ovulation is small and I'm determined to make the most of it – even if the only opportunity to do so is at a quarter to midnight on a weekday. I spent most of yesterday evening at a work event and when I finally got home was ready for bed (and not in *that* way) but according to my menstrual tracking iPhone app it was time to get down to business. Tom had tucked into two bottles of wine with the neighbour, which was a bad sign, but he greeted me with raised eyebrows and enquired if it was 'sexy time'.

I replied in the affirmative and we got to work. Asked what I wanted, I told him not to worry about warming the engine tonight and just get on with it, which he duly did. The alcohol, however, proved to inhibit his performance so I recommended he gave himself a hand, if you catch my drift.

"Just pop it back in when you're ready," I added… except he didn't!

"What did you do that for?!" I exclaimed incredulously.

"What?"

"You were supposed to do it inside me. You've wasted it now."

"Sorry, I didn't realise you were using me as a stud animal."

"What, you thought I just wanted sex at midnight?"

"Yes! You said you wanted 'sexy time' – I thought you were horny."

"No silly, I think I'm ovulating."

"Well I didn't know, did I? You have to tell me."

To be honest I'd thought it was obvious by the way I'd so readily agreed to late night nookie, but I had to concede my communication could have been clearer. It didn't stop me sulking though.

"We could have missed our one chance, we'll have to wait till next month now," I bemoaned. Poor Tom.

"I promise never to waste it again," he said earnestly, adding after a short pause "unless you're not here to put it in, that is…"

Well, I guess I can't argue with that!

October 5

It must be my age, but it seems like everyone is either getting married or having babies (and we're no exception, of course). Consequently, we spent the lovely sunny weekend visiting friends and their little ones or their ever-growing bumps, dragging Tom's 11-year-old daughter, Rosie, with us

Unlike me when I was her age, she's absolutely brilliant with small children and they simply adore her. She's told us before she'd like another brother or sister (she has a six-year-old brother via her mum and stepdad) and the babyfest got her back on the topic of siblings once again.

"So, Hannah's pregnant, Zoe's pregnant, Sarah's pregnant, Nina's pregnant and Becky's pregnant, aren't you feeling a bit left out?" she asked me, hitting the proverbial nail on the head, as she has a tendency to do.

It goes without saying that I'm delighted for them all, particularly as some of them have been trying for a very long time, but it's hard to take your mind off getting pregnant when every week another couple calls to share their happy news.

Rosie raised the subject again later.

"Are you and Daddy planning to have a baby soon, then?" she ventured over a plate of chips.

It was a difficult one, because Tom and I had agreed not to declare openly that we were trying, to avoid bringing additional stress and pressure to the situation. However, I wanted her to know it was our intention and also that baby making could be a complicated business. So I answered her honestly.

"We hope to, but it doesn't always happen straight away, you know."

"I know," she said, but seemed pleased nonetheless.

And I was too. However long it takes, it's great to know our baby has such a wonderful big sister awaiting his or her arrival.

October 10

"So, do you feel a little bit pregnant yet?" Tom asks me hopefully.

I think about it for a moment:

"Hmm I don't think so."

...But, then again, I'm not really sure what it would feel like.

Friends have told me that the first indications can be sore boobs and crampy pains in the groin (caused by the fertilised egg embedding itself in the womb), but equally this could just be a sign that your period is on its way, so not that much help.

In films, the neon-lit sign that a character is pregnant is when she starts spewing up, but in reality morning sickness might not kick in until around week six – or you might be one of the lucky ones and not suffer from morning sickness at all. So all you can really do then is wait.

It's a frustrating time, and not just for the obvious reasons. I have always enjoyed shrugging off the stresses of the working week with a healthy drink, but while there's a chance you could be pregnant it would be irresponsible to indulge in any more than a couple. Having to hold back makes it all the more disappointing when your period arrives and you realise it was all for nothing. If I can't be pregnant at least let me be drunk!! While the risk of damaging your unborn baby is never worth it, I did cover a fascinating story recently about a woman who didn't know she was pregnant until she went into labour – one week overdue as it turns out.

Apparently, she had thought she was putting on a bit of weight so had recently joined a gym. She had been carrying on as normal; drinking, eating all the things you shouldn't, but happily the baby, a little girl, was perfectly healthy.

I've got to say I find it hard to believe anyone can carry a baby to full term and not know about it – what about the kicks in the ribs, swollen ankles or massive bump?!

I've not known a women in her third trimester who hasn't been uncomfortably aware of her condition at all times. Perhaps she was in denial, who knows?

Anyway, I'm due on this Wednesday, so this month's wait will shortly be over. If I've not been successful, I will be commiserating with several large glasses of rosé.

THE FIRST TRIMESTER

October 14

So…how to put this…I am, it would appear, pregnant!!

Friday night (two days late according to my iPhone app) I decided to do a test. Tom was still on his way home after collecting Rosie for the weekend, so I had the house to myself. I peed into a pink plastic thermos mug and dipped the stick in with trepidation. I replaced the cap and placed it on the side, watching the digital display flash. The answer came quickly: 'Pregnant'.

I looked at it, looked away, looked again, looked closer, picked it up, put it down, held it under the light. I wasn't misreading it! With shaky hands and in a somewhat robotic manner, I started clearing away the pot of wee, empty packet and used test stick. I put the digital holder back in the drawer and went into the kitchen, stood trance like for a few minutes, then went back to the drawer just to check the reading one more time. I couldn't get my head round what had just happened. I'd convinced myself it would be negative.

I was supposed to be cooking spaghetti bolognaise for the family but, as if suffering from a head injury, I just couldn't work out how to do it. I guess it was the shock. I needed to speak to someone.

I texted Anna: "just did a digital test and it said 'pregnant'!" No sooner had I pressed 'send' when the phone started ringing. I answered to her screaming in my ear:

"Oh my god, oh my god is it true? Why didn't you call me?!"

Shortly followed by "So, how are you going to tell him?"

It was a good question. I didn't want to just come out and say it, and it was a bit awkward with Rosie around.

"I could text him?" I suggested.

"No you cannot!" Anna told me firmly.

"It's got to be something good. Why don't you stuff a jumper up your top and tell him he better get used to you looking like that?"

"Hmm not so sure about that one. How about I spell it out in spaghetti at dinner?"

"Whatever you do you've got to let me know his reaction. Hee hee, I'm so excited! I'm going to be the first one to babysit, okay?"

I felt better after the call and managed to get the dinner on. Then, seeing our wedding photo album poking out of my bag, I had a great idea. It had only been delivered to my office that morning so Tom was yet to see it. I found a pink Post-it note and a silver pen and wrote 'I'm Pregnant!'. I placed the note on the last page of the book – a photo of Tom and I having our first dance.

I took the book and placed it on his pillow, under the duvet. I didn't know how I was going to get through the evening without saying anything. Thankfully, Tom presented Rosie with an early 12th birthday present - a snazzy new laptop - the setting up and admiring of which provided a good distraction. As we approached 10.30pm and Tom's eyelids began to droop I counted down the minutes until he decided to head to bed. I tried to read a book as he brushed his teeth but the words failed to go in.

My heart was thumping as he pulled back the duvet and revealed the book.

"What a lovely surprise," he said.

"That's nothing!" I thought.

My mouth was dry as he made his way nearer to the end of the book.

"Hurry up!" I longed to shout, but he was lovingly inspecting every photo.

I held my breath as he began to turn the last page. He dropped the book as he saw it, covering his eyes with his hands as tears began to come.

"Oh my god, really?" he asked. I nodded. "Wow. You could have told me in the morning. I'm never going to sleep now!"

October 16 - Week 5

Still not quite able to believe it, I took another test yesterday – this time one with a 'conception indicator' feature. It confirmed that I did indeed have a bun in the oven and that I'd been cooking it for three+ weeks. In medical terms, this makes me five+ weeks pregnant; slightly further along than I'd expected – and ironically, already pregnant when I started writing this diary!

My last two cycles had been 34 days long so I'd estimated that I would ovulate on the 20th day – but that was just over two weeks ago, not three. I counted back a further week in my diary and looked for the last time we'd made love around that date.

To my horror it was at a down at heel Travelodge in Gants Hill, Essex, the morning after a friend's wedding. It really was the least salubrious place, with paper-thin walls and furnishings reminiscent of a borstal. We'd only ended up there because hubby dearest had accidentally booked (and paid for) the hotel we were meant to be staying in for the wrong date.

We had laughed, as we lay there post-coital, that if we'd just conceived and were to name the child after where it was conceived, like Posh and Becks' son Brooklyn, it would have to be Travelodge, Essex or perhaps Gants. None of which are likely to set a child up very well. Let's hope we can think of some more appealing options!

Meanwhile, I have purchased my first pregnancy book and learned that the little life form inside of me is currently the size of a sultana. Tom had a word with the sultana last night and told it: "I want you to hurry up and grow into a grape, then an apple, then a melon – first a honeydew melon and then a great big water melon!"

Maybe if it's a girl we'll call her Melanie…

October 23 - Week 6

I've spent the last few days in a constant state of worry. The thing is I just don't 'feel' pregnant. If it weren't for my missed period and positive tests I wouldn't know anything was amiss at all. There's been no morning sickness, no sore boobs, no extreme tiredness or even any constipation.

My baby book says feeling sick is caused by high levels of the pregnancy hormone hCG, which caused me to worry about having low hCG levels and the implications that might have.

I turned to the internet for reassurance and apparently it is 'normal' not to feel sick and I should be grateful, but I'm not – it's funny, I never thought I'd want to feel sick but I need to know something's going on in there!

The internet can be a source of comfort but it can also be a cause for great alarm. Having read that pregnant women should not take multi-vitamins containing vitamin A, and then discovering that the ones I'd been taking did, I anxiously Googled the risks.

The first page to be returned was an article from the Daily Mail. This is what it said:

Expectant mothers who take multi-vitamin supplements could be causing handicaps in their unborn children, it has emerged. A study by Trading Standards watchdogs and charity BDF (Birth Defects Foundation) Newlife has found that a third of all multi-vitamin suppliers do not label their products with warnings stating that they contain vitamin A, which can lead to horrific health defects. BDF Newlife chief executive, Sheila Brown, said women should avoid vitamin A like the plague.

"Horrific birth defects". Bloody hell, reading that alone could cause one to miscarry! I urgently scoured the internet for more reliable sources and found that foetuses are only at an increased risk of suffering birth defects if the mother is consuming at least four times the recommended daily allowance of vitamin A. This steadied my heart rate, but I did go on to look at which foods are rich in vitamin A, just in case there was a chance I'd exceeded the recommended daily allowance...who knows?

On top of this, I've been worrying about inadvertently eating brie or pâté and contracting listeria, or salmonella from an undercooked egg. It would appear that an embryo must navigate a veritable minefield to emerge unscathed as a healthy baby.

According to statistics, 15-20 per cent of all pregnancies will end in miscarriage in the first 12 weeks, with the risk reducing to 3-5 per cent once the foetal heartbeat can be heard.

I'm six weeks today. I just hope I can hold on for a few more precarious weeks. At least I have my first antenatal appointment next Thursday, when I shall be able to offload some of my worries.

October 31 - Week 7

I never thought I'd say this, but I'm actually quite enjoying not drinking. When I first discovered I was pregnant I'd wondered how I'd get through nine months and beyond without a drink, particularly as the industry I work in is a very social one, with frequent evening functions.

Last weekend, work afforded Tom and I the opportunity to stay in Brighton, and this would usually have meant a big Saturday night out. Instead, I attended the welcome drinks reception on Friday and partook of only cranberry juice and sparking water, pretending to have a big thirst on, before returning clear-headed to the hotel.

The following morning we rose early, determined to make the most of the day. We met up with my brother and some old friends for coffee, discovered the splendours of the Prince Regent's Pavilion and enjoyed fish and chips at Harry Ramsden's. We even found time for a spot of shopping – purchasing baby's first outfit; a super-cute panda babygrow and hat set. I know some might see it as tempting fate, but I just couldn't help myself. At this stage it's so hard to believe I have a baby inside of me, having something tangible to look at and feel is actually quite reassuring.

In the evening, we went to a comedy show at The Dome Theatre, where we tutted disapprovingly at irritating drunk people in the audience, and afterwards we took a bracing stroll on the pier, munching on sugared doughnuts. We were in bed by 11pm.

"What's happened to us?!" we cried in the morning, but we revelled in the novelty of tucking into a hearty breakfast, unaccompanied by the oh-so-familiar post-drink waves of nausea. "Look at everyone's bleary eyes!" Tom observed smugly.

Give it another week, and it will probably be the longest time I've gone without a drink since I was 15, when my friend Gemma introduced me to Bacardi in a field in Ireland.

I thought optimistically today that it might even be the start of a completely teetotal future, but perhaps I'll come back to you on that in a few more weeks…

November 6 - Week 8

We decided not to make a public announcement about the pregnancy until after the 12 week scan, and we know all is well, but we have shared the news with a few close friends, Rosie and our parents.

My father's response was to remind me about a contract I had drawn up and signed when I was 12, pledging never to get married or have a baby. Whoops, I seem to have broken both promises in the space of six months! I asked Dad if he would be launching proceedings against me for breach of contract, but he said he wouldn't – he'd just give me the document in a frame on the birth of the baby!

My mum asked anxiously if I'd been suffering with morning sickness. Apparently she was sick throughout all of her four pregnancies. Thank god I've avoided that so far.

Tom's mum jumped up and down with excitement when we told her to start preparing the top layer of our wedding cake - she's been hopefully retaining it in the freezer ready for a christening.

Rosie heard the commotion and came into the kitchen to see what it was all about. She, too, was thrilled.

"I'm going to be a sister!" she beamed. "Make it a baby girl please!"

After all the hugs and kisses, Tom's mum stood back to appraise me.

"You're not showing yet but you do look more busty, dear!" she declared.

I didn't realise she'd been keeping such a close eye on my bra size!

The first appointment with my GP was uneventful but reassuring. The doctor listened to all my worries and put my mind at rest, although I was surprised I wasn't given another pregnancy test, just to confirm. Apparently my word is good enough. She registered me on the system and gave me the forms to apply for free prescriptions and dental work. The benefits even extend to a year after birth – result! I should be pregnant more often!

I have my 'booking in' appointment with the midwife at the hospital this

Saturday. I'm told they will be taking my blood. I am trying not to think about this as I have a big phobia of the red stuff. I've never had a blood test before and I'm worried I will pass out and/or be sick, like the time my friend pricked my finger for a diabetes test.

Don't even mention the birth. Looks like I'm going to have to 'man up'…

November 13 - Week 9

The blood test went surprisingly well…the bit afterwards, not so much. I had kept my eyes closed throughout and didn't feel any more than a scratch, as the kind nurse had promised.

"That wasn't too bad", I thought gratefully, but my relief was short-lived. As I stood to leave that familiar combination of dizziness, pins and needles and nausea set in and soon enough Tom had enlisted the help of another prospective father to carry me back to the bed.

"You are very pale," commented the nurse, "perhaps you're anaemic?"

If I am at least I will find out now. They also check you for syphilis and HIV (yikes, hope I'm okay on that front!) and find out your blood type.

Unfortunately the blood testing is far from over; I have to have another one next Sunday to check the baby for Downs' syndrome, and then there are several more tests to be done as the pregnancy progresses.

The 'booking in' appointment, as it is known, also involved the midwife asking lots of questions about mine and Tom's family health history. Because my dad has diabetes and high blood pressure these are things which will have to be monitored on me. And because I had asthma as a child, this will also have to be monitored – apparently it is one of the conditions that can be exacerbated by pregnancy.

I didn't get to see the maternity ward, as I had hoped, although tours can be arranged. When the GP asked me which hospital I wanted I simply chose the nearest, but I have since searched the internet for reviews and read some worrying feedback, so I was really hoping to put my mind at rest.

What disturbs me the most is that you probably won't meet your midwife for the birth until the day itself. I am concerned about being treated as just another faceless woman who needs to be processed as quickly as possible to free up the bed.

I had seriously been considering requesting a caesarean. I figured that at least this way I would maintain some degree of control and not be brutally ripped apart with forceps or left in labour in the waiting room. But having visited the hospital, I'm not sure I want to go there at all.

I can't believe I'm saying this, having always been an advocate for all possible pain relief and medical intervention, but I'm now seriously considering a home birth. The luxury of my own bed, my husband with me at all times and the attention of a dedicated midwife is becoming increasingly appealing. I think it's something I might look into…

November 21 - Week 10

I had my second appointment at the hospital today; to pick up my blood test results and give them some more of my precious ruby nectar for the combined Down's syndrome test. I'm pleased to report that I do not have HIV, syphilis, an iron deficiency or any other problem! I also found out that I am A+ (at least my blood gets high grades!). I managed not to faint this time, too.

Just two more weeks to go now until the 12-week scan. Despite being very excited, this week has seen the return of the worrywart. I'm so paranoid that they'll tell me there's no heartbeat and everything will be over. It happened to a close friend of mine. The doctor told her she'd lost the baby at about eight weeks but she didn't start to bleed until after the scan. The only indication she'd had was the disappearance of her morning sickness.

I haven't had much of that, but I have been having to get up twice nightly for toilet trips and my boobs have been tender, so I guess they are all good signs. I've certainly put on weight, too – things are starting to feel decidedly snug.

I'm going to Barcelona for a trade exhibition this week and have been trying to find items in the wardrobe that disguise my rapidly-growing paunch. However, I have now told my editor I'm pregnant, so that's a weight off my mind. I thought it best, just in case I'm expected to stay out late drinking, plus I'm going to have to leave work early for my scan on the 5th. She seemed genuinely pleased and excited for me, despite the inconvenience my absence will inevitably cause.

I can't wait until I have the A-Okay to tell everyone. There are still some of my closest friends who don't know, but that's more because I want to wait to see them face-to-face, rather than tell them over the phone.

We did let on to one friend this weekend, who joined us when we took Rosie and her friend ice-skating. I sat the skating out with a hot chocolate for fear of falling over, so we had to offer some explanation. After enthusiastically congratulating us she leaned in conspiratorially and whispered, "So am I!"

She will be due in July, a month after me. This means that we have friends expecting babies every month from now to July. Do you think there's something in the water?

November 28 - Week 11

My editor may have taken news of my pregnancy well, but my managing director is a different matter entirely.

Having just been informed that one of my colleagues would not be returning to work from maternity leave, he told the team that any new members of staff would have to be sterile! I giggled, wondering if he was also having a dig at me, but my editor said, no, she was yet to tell him. “Oh dear, that’s really not going to go down well then, is it?” I said. She grimaced in reply.

She was scheduled to meet with him the following morning, so said she would do it then.

“What did he say?” I asked eagerly afterwards.

“It went something like this: ‘oh fuck’,” she revealed. He had also confirmed that my replacement would be a man.

I wasn’t looking forward to seeing him, but when we did bump into each other I got no more response than a small nod of recognition. Later that day we were stood next to each other but he seemed to be acting as if I was not there.

I told my editor how strangely he was acting. “I thought he might at least say congratulations,” I admitted. It turned out that he was apparently waiting for me to tell him myself, but I said I would not. He knows I know he knows – if you know what I mean? Why do I need to inform him personally? He should say something to me!

Anyway, I’m not going to lose any sleep over it. After my scan next week I’ll hopefully by able to announce it officially and put a stop to this silliness.

December 6 - Week 12

We saw our baby for the first time yesterday. We saw her eyes and nose and little hands and feet. The scan image was crystal clear; it really was the most incredible thing I’ve ever seen.

“You have a textbook baby,” the sonographer told us as she measured her up – six centimetres top to bottom, making her 12 weeks and four days and due on June 14. We heard her heartbeat, which was good and strong, and listened to my blood whooshing around. Baby was wriggling all over the place, rolling over, waving.

“You’ve got a live wire there,” said the sonographer.

Perhaps baby knew we were looking and was just showing off?!

I’m referring to the baby as ‘her’ because that’s my feeling, but the sonographer told us it was too early to tell. Apparently, the penis and the clitoris are the same size at this stage – interesting! I'm desperate to know, though. I'm so convinced it's a girl, I very naughtily bought a gorgeous little summer dress and sun hat, which were in the sale. If it is actually a boy I need to get my head round that, lest I start dressing him in pink and putting ribbons in his hair!

Anna says her friend paid for a private early sexing scan and this is something I might look into. For now, I'm just so happy and relieved that everything is looking good and we can finally start sharing the news!

THE SECOND TRIMESTER

December 10 – Week 13

Ok, so I know I said finding out the sex of my unborn child wasn't the most important thing right now, but I lied.

I found myself up late, looking at pictures on the internet which show how the angle of the 'nubbin' indicate whether it's a boy or a girl. Studying my scan images, at first I thought "it's a girl!" but when I looked closer at the 'angle of the dangle' I thought "no, it's a boy!". As a result I really didn't sleep well that night and vowed to get booked in for an early gender scan the next day.

Unless you want to pay £500, most of the clinics won't offer the service before 16 weeks – for me, this milestone falls on December 29. I thought I'd have to wait until after New Year, but I found a company called Ultrasound Direct in Richmond, which has availability on December 31. Quite some way to mark New Year's Eve, I think you'll agree!

Tom's initial reaction was "God, you're soooo impatient!", but he now agrees it is a good idea to find out in case our conviction it's a girl turns out to be wrong.

I saw Anna last night and asked her to tell me all the great things about having a boy (she has two).

"They're much easier," she said "and more affectionate," but she was also pulling a face at the same time, which made me doubtful.

She said the best idea was to get her 'psychic' two-year-old daughter to give me a prediction.

"She's been right twice before," she told me earnestly.

So we called her over and asked her whether the baby in my tummy was a little girl or a little boy.

"Little girl," she answered confidently.

We asked her again an hour later and she repeated her affirmation. Perhaps I could have saved myself £79 on the scan? At least we won't have to wait very long to find out…

December 15 – Week 14

There were only two people I was anxious about telling news of my pregnancy – ironically my two oldest friends.

Gemma and Elle have always been 'anti-kids' and both tried to talk me out of trying to get pregnant when I announced my plan earlier in the year.

"'You're too young, you'll ruin your life," they said.

"I'm not some clueless teenager," I insisted. "I'm 30, I'm married and I've thought about it very seriously."

I think the issue is that *they're* not ready for me to have a child. They're scared of our group dynamic changing and I do sympathise with that. Things will inevitably change, but not necessarily for the worse I believe.

With Elle's hen do approaching I knew I'd have to spill the beans soon, but couldn't find the right moment. Strangely it was taken out of my hands, when Elle called me and demanded:

"Are you pregnant?"

"No, what makes you say that?" I flustered.

Apparently, she was washing her face when she suddenly had an overwhelming feeling about it and had to call immediately (she's always been a little weird like that).

I finally admitted that I was and after an initial 'oh no' she actually took it pretty well and said as long as I was happy, so was she. We decided to wait and tell Gemma when we went to stay with her in Ireland for Elle's hen do. That was last weekend.

Gemma sat quietly and digested the news. Her boyfriend scolded her for not congratulating me, which she eventually did – if through gritted teeth! Surprisingly Elle even helped put a positive spin on it, saying they'd be bound to love the baby like a niece or nephew because it was part of me.

Thankfully the revelation didn't put a dampener on the evening. Gemma fixed me a non-alcoholic cocktail and we got on with the fun and laughter. In a quieter moment, Gemma admitted seeing my scan picture had unearthed some confusing feelings surrounding two terminations she'd had in the past, and she spoke about her fear of everybody having kids and leaving her behind.

I actually think me having this baby might help both Gemma and Elle to confront their issues around children. Either that or I am ruining my life and they shall be proved right…

December 22 – Week 15

We've come to the conclusion that with the baby coming we'll need to move house – or at least I have anyway. Tom has been dead set against leaving London and finding somewhere cheaper in the suburbs, but besides the need to save a bit of cash, I just can't see how we're all going to fit into our two-bedroom flat. Our second bedroom is Tom's office (he works from home as a marketing consultant) and it doubles up as Rosie's room when she comes to stay every fortnight. It also houses our wardrobes, the ironing board, cross trainer (upon which we hang more clothes) and all the other random junk that won't fit anywhere else. So, you get the picture. It's all very well that the baby will be sharing with us initially, but what about the pram, nursing chair, baby rocker, play mat etc. etc.? Babies may be small but they sure take up a lot of space.

Thankfully a recent visit by Rosie and her friend and all the mess that comes with tweenage girls helped Tom come round to my way of thinking. In fact he was pretty much pulling his hair out, and when I showed him a three-bedroom house to rent for the same price as our flat he agreed: "we need to move, don't we."

Once I had his blessing, I got immediately to work and booked a viewing. I went to see it last night after work, as it's only 10 miles from my office in Sussex. It's a townhouse in an old converted mental institution and it's huge! It has two bathrooms, high ceilings, on-site communal gym/pool and lovely country views. Plus it's right next to the hospital – handy given the current circumstances! I knew we'd have to snap it up quick so called Tom and gave him an aural show round. He agreed we should go for it. Excitedly, we got in touch with the agent first thing this morning. While we knew moving was going to be an expense, we weren't expecting to be charged a £300 referencing fee by the lettings agency on top of having to shell out a month and a half's rent as a deposit. Then we found out some of the white goods listed on the particulars would not be coming with the house. Tom went into 'man mode' playing hardball with the negotiations.

They were back and forth all day and then things went quiet. Never a good sign.

"I think I might have blown it," he told me.

It turns out that the landlord has indeed decided to go with another interested party. Tom is gutted. I'm so disappointed, but trying not to show it. I know he was only trying to save us money.

I just want to get settled before I get any bigger and start getting our home ready for baby. The nesting instinct is setting in already! This morning I'd been so happy that we could relax over Christmas knowing our moving date was set for February. Oh well, I guess I just need to get back on those property websites after the festive break. At least we are off on holiday to sunny Tenerife tomorrow, and we have something even more exciting to look forward to on our return – our gender scan! Happy Christmas everyone.

January 2 – Week 16

Drum roll please…it's a….BOY!!

So, not what we were banking on. Looks like the summer dress and hat will have to find another home. Of course, we are still delighted, but Tom and I have both had to rapidly adjust our mindsets.

It didn't come as a complete shock. While we were away we both dreamed about our baby being a boy (although, worryingly, in one of my dreams it was a male Alsatian puppy?!). Then Elle (who I now firmly believe is a witch) called the day before and said she had also dreamed we were having a boy and I was pretty sure she'd be proven right. Indeed, there was no doubting our little one's sex; "and you can clearly see there's the willy," said the sonographer.

"I can; it's quite a big one!" I replied.

We went and sat in a coffee shop afterwards to digest the news. "Our son," we repeated to each other, trying it on for size. Then we headed off to buy our first blue baby bits. We found a cute little spotty babygrow and a farm animal mobile for the nursery and were soon getting used to the idea.

"I can still do things like baking and painting and horse riding with him, can't I?" I asked, suddenly seeing weekends spent standing at the side of a muddy football pitch.

"Of course you can, honey. You can do all the things you would have done with a daughter, apart from maybe dollies and dresses," Tom reassured me.

And I know it will be wonderful; lots of my friends have little boys who they simply adore. I think it's just that we had only planned to have one child and it all seems very final. While we have Rosie in our lives, she's very close to her mum (as she should be) and, at 12, is no longer a little girl. I couldn't help thinking about how I'll never pass on my wedding dress or share any of those other precious mother-daughter moments.

"Maybe we could have just one more?" I ventured.

"And that's how we'll end up with three boys!" Tom replied, referring to a prediction made by a fortune teller when I was 15. He's probably right.

My mum laughed knowingly when I told her the news.

"I knew it was a boy when you said the baby was wriggling all over the place at the 12 week scan; that's boys all over!"

And she should know, she's had three of them. Incidentally, three boys who, between them, have brought such a lot of trouble and heartache, which I guess is another reason I have reservations.

I don't want it to sound like I'm not excited. I am, very. And now I know who's inside I'm sure me and my boy will grow closer every day. Tom and I have even settled on a name (we did have a shortlist for both sexes, despite being convinced we were having a girl), which makes my little boy bump even more real. I can't think of a better way to kick off the New Year!

January 9 – Week 17

I have a real case of the January blues. First week of the year and everything is going wrong. First, my tenant couldn't pay his rent causing me to exceed my already massive overdraft and leaving me with NO money, and then Tom gets a nasty surprise from the Inland Revenue.

Turns out he owes a lot more tax than he expected for last year (the year he started his own company) and also needs to start making payments on account for the current year.

This comes at a time when we are facing the additional expense of a house move and an impending new arrival. All a little bit overwhelming. Can I go back to bed please?

To be honest, my finances are in a parlous state and I will very soon have to contact my loan and credit card providers to tell them I can no longer afford my repayments. I'd been hoping to put it off until I started maternity leave to give me the option of borrowing some money to help me with my own planned business start-up, but I don't think I have a choice. It's horrible to be worrying about this when I should be enjoying the excitement of being 17 weeks pregnant. Instead of thinking about feeling baby's first kicks, I'm fretting over how we will afford the pram and cot.

People often say 'money doesn't make you happy' and I know this is true but it's also true that having no money can make you unhappy.

Money worries are the only thing in my life that make me unhappy, everything else is pretty much perfect, so I guess I must count my blessings for that.

Tom says that the hard times make him appreciate the good ones even more. I just hope it's not too long until good times start coming our way!

January 16 – Week 18

Well, what a difference a week makes. I have been extremely proactive, finding us somewhere to live and taking the first steps to get my debts under control.

We've found a lovely three-bedroom cottage with a tranquil garden that looks onto trees and fields – an ideal location for raising the little one, and it's right around the corner from where I work. Best of all, it's being rented by a private landlord which means we avoid the hefty 'referencing fees' and only have to put down four weeks deposit instead of six. We even managed to get £50 off the rent!

I finally undertook the task I'd been putting off for so long; calculating all of my debts and outgoings. All in all, I owe a shocking £25k – yikes! Before you label me financially irresponsible, this is debt which has been building up for more than 10 years and has been compounded by a business failure, various vehicle nightmares, the housing market crash…and just a little bit of retail therapy.

Anyway I got in touch with the debt charity Step Change and discussed my options. They are recommending an IVA (individual voluntary agreement), which is basically an alternative to bankruptcy. Agreements would be made with my creditors regarding how much I could afford to repay each month and then, after a period of five years, any remaining debt would be written off. It does mean my credit rating would be shot to pieces, and there are some implications for the equity in my flat, but at least this way there would be an end in sight. It would certainly feel as if an incredible burden had been lifted from my shoulders.

The other option is to write to each creditor individually, requesting reduced payments and a freeze on interest until such time as I am back at work and can afford to make full payments again. If they are willing to do this (which I'm told they usually are), it won't hurt my credit rating so much and my flat will remain safe, but it does mean the debt won't 'go away'.

So, I just need to think it all through fully and decide which option is best for me. However, prior to any action I have taken the opportunity to purchase a travel system pram from Mothercare (reduced from £400 to £200) on my credit card. I know it's naughty but making sure baby is provided for is a priority – and to be fair it was a vastly more economical choice than the £1,000 Bugaboo prams I have been salivating over online.

In other news, I am now 18 weeks pregnant and still waiting eagerly to feel baby's first kick!

January 23 – Week 19

There are lots of medications that should be avoided in pregnancy, but you may be surprised to hear that pregnant women should not even smell Vicks. Suffering with a stinking cold last week, I learned that all I could take to relive my misery was paracetamol – not even inhaling eucalyptus is allowed, the pharmacist informed me.

Just to compound matters, we were on deadline at work, putting the February issue of the magazine to bed, so I was unable to take it easy in bed. I was proofing pages until my head felt ready to explode. Needless to say, I was feeling pretty sorry for myself. But to give Tom his due, he did his best to look after me; having dinner on the table when I got home, driving me to the station and dishing out back rubs. I don't know if it's the pregnancy hormones or just that I was tired and ill, but I felt particularly emotional this week; bursting into floods of tears at random moments, like watching 'One Born Every Minute'.

"What's wrong?" Tom asked concerned. And all I could sob was:

"I don't know" – and I really didn't.

In among all the gratuitous tissue use last week, something amazing did happen. I felt my baby move for the first time. I was lying in bed and I felt three little jabs low in my groin. I put my hand there to investigate and actually felt movement beneath it! It is an odd sensation, but almost like a pulse or an internal twinge.

This weekend I was able to share notes with one of Tom's friends who gave birth six weeks ago and another who is 30 weeks pregnant. Sarah had a beautiful baby girl, but endured a very arduous birth – during which the hospital caught on fire! She filled me in on some of less pleasant aspects of early motherhood, such as the six weeks of menstruation after birth and the ridiculously leaky boobs.

We also heard the happy news that yet another couple in our social circle is expecting, which takes the total up to nine! While last year was weddings and 30th birthdays, it seems the next two will be full of christenings and first birthdays. What a great adventure this thing we call life is…

January 28 – 20 weeks

Baby is very well travelled considering he's only 20 weeks old – he's been to Dublin, Barcelona, Tenerife and, this week, Budapest. I don't think he made much of the beautiful architecture and view of the Danube but he did seem to have a very strong reaction to a Hungarian orchestra.

I was in the city for a work conference, which culminated with a wonderful gala dinner at a railway museum in a former train depot. We were treated to a rousing performance of classical music, which had baby vigorously kicking along throughout – I've got to say, I was quite relieved when it was over!

My bump must be getting bigger now because somebody noticed it for the first time and asked if I was expecting. Always a risky question, I think! I was happy because even to me it just looks like I over-indulged a bit at Christmas.

I took advantage of the exchange rate to pick up a few baby bargains in Zara, including an adorable pair of cord dungarees, a little checked shirt and a hat and gloves for next winter. They were so cute I didn't even feel a pang of disappointment walking past the dresses. Neither did I feel the need to buy anything for myself, I told Tom proudly.

"Yes, but it is really for you, isn't it – he's inside you," he replied, but I felt less guilty for spending anyway…

Tom got to feel baby kick for the first time last night and is hopeful he has a champion footballer in the making. He's certainly tearing up the turf in there, resulting in rather unpleasant acid reflux for me. It feels like I have a burning lump in my throat, and is particularly bad when I lie down at night. One of the many joys of motherhood, I guess.

Tomorrow is a big day – we move house and I have my 21-week scan. Not ideal timing but I wanted to get it done before being transferred to the new hospital and possibly having to wait a few more weeks. I'm looking forward to having another peek in the sunroof and seeing just what he's up to in there!

February 11 – Week 22

Well, what a hectic two weeks since my last diary entry! We had our final scan, moved house, forensically cleaned the old one, got snowed in, sold a sofa, bought a sofa, painted walls, put up pictures, had an epic Ikea trip, put flat-pick furniture together, entertained Rosie over the half-term and I put in the extra hours at work getting a bumper anniversary edition of the magazine to bed – I'm exhausted just typing it!

I'm only glad I've entered what they call the 'nesting phase' and been able to tap hidden energy reserves. I must say getting up this morning was quite a struggle, though. Still, I now live just a short walk from my office, which affords me an extra hour in bed – heaven!

We're really settling into the new place now and relishing the extra space (as are our two cats!). Baby has his very own room and as we speak Tom is going to fetch a Mamas and Papas cot and changing table I bought on eBay for just £60.

I have a beautiful wall sticker of kittens playing in a tree, which I intend to put up over the weekend and Tom wants to set up the baby monitor "so we can use it as a walkie talky when I'm downstairs and you're upstairs," apparently.

I've also finally put the pram together, which had been languishing in a box in a cupboard at work for weeks. It's quite a lot bigger than I'd hoped for and we can't work out how to fold it down yet, but it looks nice and comfy.

Baby continues to have nightly parties in my tummy, but stubbornly refused to uncross his legs when I went for the scan. The sonographer said it was lucky I already knew the sex because she wouldn't have been able to tell me. Shyness aside, everything else looked good with him and he's measuring up nicely, despite my modest bump.

I'm sad that I won't get another chance to see him until he makes his first public appearance, but as long as he keeps up the sucker punches I'll know he's there and everything's okay.

Now, I'm off for a well-deserved evening of relaxation; dinner, a DVD and an early night.

February 18 – Week 23

I wish I could tell you I'm blooming, but some unpleasant pregnancy side effects have emerged this week.

I won't beat around the bush; I've got a haemorrhoid. A little fleshy pea-sized lump. Sorry, too much information, I know.

Apparently it's very common in pregnancy, caused by the weight of the baby on your interior bits and exacerbated by constipation – another common pregnancy complaint. Thankfully it's not causing me any discomfort but it is a little embarrassing.

Also embarrassing, is the fact that I've started snoring. According to Tom, it's become a nightly occurrence and twice this week he's been forced to sleep in the spare room.

I told him just to give me a shove and last night I was aware of him tapping me on the head a couple of times.

"But I wasn't snoring," I insisted in the morning.

"No, you were making other weird noises, sort of grunting," he informed me. How very attractive…

Truth be told, I've also been a bit windy too. Oh, poor Tom!

On a more wholesome note, some friends of ours, Emily and Simon, welcomed a beautiful baby girl into the world on the weekend. She was born at home, under the guidance of a yoga-teaching doula and Emily and Simon have since been singing the praises of the 'hypnobirthing' approach.

To be honest, they seem to have gone a little bit hippy, preaching about the wonders of a 'drug-free natural birthing experience' but it has convinced me to plan for a home birth, too. It's a big decision to step away from the reassuring facilities of a hospital, but if birth is a natural process perhaps we medicalise it unnecessarily? By choosing to give birth at home, I won't need to worry about the bumpy 30-minute journey to hospital through country lanes, I'll have two midwives in attendance focused solely on me, and, if anything does go wrong I can be transferred via ambulance.

Emily gave birth in an inflatable birthing pool and said the warm water was a great natural pain reliever, so I'm going to look into getting one myself. I've also asked Anna to do the honours as my 'birth partner' (she's not much good at yoga, but she's helped out at a birth before and will be a very reassuring presence).

With regards to yoga, I'm going to enquire about local classes. All the spiritual stuff aside, it makes sense that strengthened muscles and a relaxed state of mind will aid giving birth.

The thing is, a story my friend Kate told me about her yoga class always sticks in my mind. There was a woman who always let off wind reducing the rest of the class to stifled hysterics. And if this week is anything to go by, I'm just worried that that person could be me!

February 27 – Week 24

Yesterday I celebrated my birthday. Suffice to say it was a rather tamer affair than last year, when I turned 30. Tom had turned 40 five days before and so we had a joint 70th party, with 1970s fancy dress. There was some legendary merry-making and, as I recall, we didn't make it to bed until noon the next day!

This time not a drop of alcohol passed my lips. Instead, I enjoyed a thoroughly civilised celebration, going for a spa session and afternoon tea with five girlfriends at the beautiful Alexander House Hotel in West Sussex.

I was a little disappointed to learn that, being pregnant, it wasn't advisable for me to use the Jacuzzi or sauna (in case the baby overheats), but I could indulge in a vigorous back massage from the water jets and a relaxing swim.

We were then rewarded with a fine selection of teas, little sandwiches with the crusts cut off and yummy cakes. Cake seems to have become a big part of my life (or more accurately, bigger part) since becoming pregnant. I think it must be my substitute for wine. But my increasing consumption appears to have been noted; my birthday presents included a pretty teapot and a cake stand, as well as a cupcake recipe book and cake decorating set from Rosie. The banana cupcakes look particularly delicious and will be my first project!

In other, more unsavoury news, I continue to experience new pregnancy side effects. Although I'm blaming Rosie for this one. She thought it would be funny to 'frape' her dad by posting a bogus status update on his Facebook profile.

It went like this: 'I just sneezed and a bit of wee came out!'

This caused much hilarity and prompted one of his friends to ask if he was pregnant. Anyway, this exact thing happened to me the very next day! I was out walking my friend Elle's little dog, who we're looking after while she and James are off getting married in Sri Lanka, when I sneezed and simultaneously wet myself. I was so shocked that I dropped my iPhone on the pavement! I can't believe that I have lost control of my bladder already

– I thought that sort of thing was supposed to happen after you'd had the baby? All I can say is thank God I don't suffer from hay fever…

March 3 – Week 25

Have you ever tried to contract your clitoral hood? I'm guessing probably not, unless you've been to pregnancy yoga before or had a particularly bad lover.

This was exactly what we were asked to do during my first yoga session and it's not that easy, I'll have you know!

We were also told to locate and contract our vaginal walls and anus.

"Contract those muscles, hold, then let go…totally let go," said the instructor as we all knelt down in a praying position, bottoms in the air.

Given my recent flatulence, I was praying not to 'let go'!

On top of this we were encouraged to take deep breaths and make loud groans or 'raspberry' noises as we exhaled. Honestly, it was too funny. I was so close to bursting into laughter and thanked my lucky stars that I was among strangers and not any of my friends, which would have seen me in uncontrollable hysterics.

That said, I didn't think the session was totally silly. It was very relaxing and therapeutic to focus the mind elsewhere (even on my anus) after a busy day at work. We practised 'yogic breathing', which involved drawing breath through three areas of the body; first from the abdomen to the chest and then up to the collarbone.

Nadia, the instructor said that this helps to connect us with our babies and that we might feel them moving, and I did!

I came away from the class with a sense of wellbeing and a fully flexed pelvic floor – clearly, it reaches parts other exercise classes can't! I will be returning for my second session on Thursday and am ready to grunt and groan with the best of them!

March 10 – Week 26

I was in two minds about whether to sign up for NCT antenatal classes. On the one hand I had friends who said they were a great way to meet fellow mums and potential lifelong friends, but on the other were those who thought they were a waste of time. On top of this they cost £180 – not an insubstantial amount when saving for a new arrival.

However, in the end I decided it would be a worthwhile investment if it equipped me with knowledge and support that would make the birth and early weeks of child-raising easier.

We attended our first class this week, held at a primary school a little way out of town and led by Nicki, a middle management-type mum of three. We were one of eight couples of varying ages and backgrounds. I instantly started scoping them out to see if any of them had friend potential. None of them seemed quite 'like me' but they were all very nice – and we discovered that two couples live just around the corner, which could come in handy for babysitting!

The session was certainly designed to break the ice, with the first task seeing us separated into a mum group and a dad group and asked to make a list of topics we wished to explore via the classes. The dad's list included 'how soon after birth is it safe for the woman to start exercising?', prompting reproachful looks from each woman to her partner.

"Who asked that? I bet it was you!" we all accused, but the men closed ranks and would not reveal the culprit.

Before any men vs. women fights could break out, we were regrouped into mixed-sex groups and tasked with labelling a plastic pelvis, identifying parts of the womb or organising pictures of a baby being born into the right order. If only I'd paid more attention in biology!

I was surprised to learn that the baby has to negotiate somewhat of an obstacle course in its bid for freedom. The changing width and breadth of the pelvis means the baby must swivel from front to side three times to get its shoulders through the maze. This was demonstrated with a wooden box with slits in it and a one-dimensional wooden baby on a stick known as a Dutch pelvis and Dutch baby.

Other obstacles for the child to overcome include the bladder and the bowels, which act like speed bumps if they are full.

"Dads, you need to make sure mum goes to the loo every hour, even if she doesn't feel like it," Nicki told us. Apparently, the (ever-helpful) body produces even more urine than normal during labour.

We were guided through the different stages of labour and told not to forget the acronym UFO, which stands for upright, forward and open – the best position for birthing.

Meanwhile, we should be 'rocking and rolling' our hips, causing the baby's head to rub on the cervix and help speed up active labour. In total the class spanned two and half hours and didn't finish until 10.15pm, by which time my head was spinning with all the information, but I am a firm believer in the saying 'forewarned is forearmed'. Having said that, I'm not sure anything can truly prepare one for becoming a mother. I will just have to put my faith in another mother – Mother Nature!

March 21 – Week 27

According to official consensus (among my friends and work colleagues, at least) I have finally 'popped'.

At 28 weeks tomorrow, and close to the beginning of my third trimester (otherwise known as the home stretch), baby has finally decided to clear up the question regarding my consumption of pies, and whether or not there had just been a few too many.

I am now the proud owner of a big round front bumper. Elle even made me a fabulous diamanté 'baby on board' T-shirt to celebrate.

Londoners will be familiar with the badges bearing the same slogan to be worn by expectant mothers on the tube. I had been putting off getting one until I had a decent sized bump in case anyone thought me a fraud, but I met up with a pregnant colleague at a trade show this week and she insisted I have one of her stash of five! I put it on somewhat sheepishly but the train was so tightly packed no one could see it anyway!

I'm definitely noticing a more frequent need to sit down. It often feels like the baby is using my bladder as a pillow and can make walking quite uncomfortable. I'm also getting short of breath quickly and am panting like a (very unfit) dog by the time I've climbed the hill to work.

Still, it's about the only panting I'm doing at the moment…There seems to be something getting between Tom and I these days, if you catch my drift.

Him on top is no longer an option and, although we are experimenting with new positions, we haven't yet settled on one that suits both of us. Baby has been keeping us preoccupied with other things, however. Monday was almost entirely dominated by him, which is worrying considering he's not even born yet. We had to go to the hospital to see the consultant and then have a glucose blood test. This is to check for gestational diabetes and involved drinking half a bottle of Lucozade and then having my blood taken an hour later. I should find out the results tomorrow when I see my midwife.

After the hospital, it was off to antenatal: "Do I have to come? It's soooo boring," wailed Tom.

I told him he did, as he'd helped get me into this mess. I was gratified that the session required the men to practise massage techniques on the women. Meanwhile, he was consoled by the tea and biscuits. Next week, however, there are two sessions, which might require more of an incentive. Perhaps I'd better refer to the Karma Sutra for some ideas…

March 25 – Week 28

Let's be honest, newborn babies aren't always the most attractive things. Florid, squinting and squirming – some might say it's a look only a mother could love. But even the most besotted mother might be a little concerned if their baby was to emerge covered in downy fur or with a rash of spots. It was for this reason our NCT teacher Nicki sought to educate us about common – but harmless – afflictions that could mar the appearance of our progeny.

With the aid of some delightful pictures, we learned about vernix; a waxy or cheese-like substance that can cover a baby's skin, cyanosis; which gives an alarming blue colour to the hands and feet, and crusty cradle cap – best treated with olive oil.

We were warned that we might even give birth to a Conehead (refer to the 1993 film starring Dan Akroyd), since babies' heads remain very flexible to help them squeeze through the birth canal. Thankfully, this should rectify itself within a couple of weeks.

Other ailments include sucking blisters, which appear on the baby's lip and look like a cold sore, but are actually caused by over zealous thumb sucking (God help the mother's nipples!), and milk spots – which MUST NOT be squeezed despite giving your lovely baby the complexion of a zitty teenager.

On top of this, our babies will probably be boss eyed and swollen-faced, and if they've been delivered with forceps could have all manner of painful looking abrasions.

"You'll probably be so high on oxytocin you won't even notice, but its best to be prepared in case you do," said Nicki.

Oh my poor little lad. I think I might put a ban on camera phones and let him have a chance to brush up a bit before he greets his public.

THE THIRD TRIMESTER

April 2 – Week 29

I've really been very lucky in my pregnancy so far. While others have suffered from dreadful sickness, excruciating lower back pain, uncomfortable swelling or even worrying spotting, I've pretty much sailed through, so I don't want to complain. However, this acid reflux is really starting to become a problem.

Previously an unpleasant acidy burp would wake me up once or twice a night, but the third trimester seems to have brought with it almost permanent sleep-disrupting heartburn. Apparently, this is caused by progesterone relaxing muscle tissue between the stomach and the gullet, allowing gastric acid to seep through. Yuk!

I've tried a number of remedies. Peppermint heartburn relief medicine, the gloopy consistency of which makes me gag; chewable Gaviscon tablets which taste like chalk and get stuck in my teeth; eating fresh pineapple after meals – enjoyable if not that effective – and propping myself into an almost vertical position in bed, resulting in neck and shoulder pains.

Other advice offered by pregnancy books includes eating very small meals, avoiding spicy or rich foods and cutting out chocolate. Sounds sensible, but my desire to have a good night's sleep is countered by my ferocious appetite and constant hankering for sugary treats…

At least I am now officially in my third trimester and have just a little over 10 weeks to go. In theory, anyway. My friends and I were predicting what date baby would arrive last night. One thinks baby will come on June 18 – our first wedding anniversary, another believes he will be later, on the 22nd, while I think he'll be just two days late, on the 16th.

Babies can be quite unpredictable, as demonstrated by the birth of two friends' little ones this week. Hannah and Zoe are both nurses working at the same hospital who, despite having due dates six weeks apart, ended up giving birth within 12 hours of each other. Zoe's waters broke on Friday at just 33 weeks. She was sent home with antibiotics but was back in hospital on Tuesday, just as best friend Hannah went into labour. Zoe gave birth naturally to a 5lb baby boy, while Hannah delivered a boy nearly twice the size by emergency C-section!

While neither experience was ideal, both mothers and babies are doing well and they're well placed to support each other, being just three rooms apart on the ward!

April 9 – Week 30

Funbags, boobies, jugs… our breasts go by many a comical name, but they do not exist for the soul purpose of fuelling schoolboy jokes (and fantasies). They're quite amazing, actually, as I discovered at a session on breastfeeding this week.

Before becoming pregnant, I'd felt quite indignant about the pressure put on women to breastfeed and the huge amounts of propaganda in its favour touted by our health agencies. "They're my breasts and I'll do with them as I please," I'd thought. I didn't believe the benefits for baby were that much greater than formula feeding, but now I'm coming to understand the wonderment of the white stuff.

You don't need to explain it to baby – apparently it knows to head straight for the milk bar as soon as it comes out. Just type 'breast crawl' into YouTube to witness the phenomenon. This skin-to-skin contact has a proven calming effect, slowing the baby's heart rate.

A mother's milk offers baby everything it needs for the first six months of life and helps to develop a strong immune system. Best of all, it's free, on tap, burns baby blubber and negates the need for sterilising and heating up bottles. You don't even need to wash your nipples before feeds as they're self-cleaning – clever, eh?

A baby that is breastfed suffers less wind and –allegedly – less offensive nappies. It has other uses too. Baby suffering from sticky eye discharge? Just squirt a bit of milk in it!

And breastfeeding doesn't mean dad can't get involved. Once expressed, milk keeps for 12-hours unrefrigerated or 7 days in the fridge – and as long as 6 months if frozen.

The benefits are clear (or milky, if you like) but of course it doesn't always go to plan and breastfeeding does not come naturally for every mother and baby. That I 'might not be able to do it' had been a concern, but the breastfeeding counsellor was very reassuring, stating that there are only 3 per cent of women who cannot physically do it. Problems normally result from the baby not latching on properly and she gave us advice to help make sure that it does.

She did warn us, however, that the baby will want to feed every two to three hours, taking 20 minutes to drain each breast. Images of dairy cows come to mind, but on the plus side, she said that feeding is the best time to enjoy a glass of wine. Although I think I may need more than a glass to tolerate a baby attached to my breasts ten times a day!

April 15 – Week 31

I've started to worry again recently. It was something Elle's mum said. I'm sure she meant well but it's just given me something else to stress about. She told me I should get checked for a bacteria commonly carried in the vagina, which can be passed on to the baby during birth, sometimes causing serious illness or even death. I'd never heard of it before, it's not in any of my pregnancy books and I'm not aware of any routine screening for it, but according to a Google search a quarter of women carry Group B streptococcus (GBS) in their vaginas. And the really worrying thing about it is it doesn't have any obvious symptoms.

Luckily I had a midwife check up this week and was able to get some more information. I asked her why GBS wasn't tested for if it is so common and potentially life threatening to newborns. She said that although the bacteria could be passed to the baby, it doesn't usually lead to an infection – only around 340 babies a year in the UK develop complications. And because GBS comes and goes there's no point testing for it prior to labour. I didn't find it 100 per cent reassuring and asked whether I should buy a home testing kit. She said I should if it would put my mind at rest, but it would probably be a waste of money given the bacteria's transience – if I have it now, it doesn't mean I'll have it in nine week's time.

Having thought about it, I've decided she's probably right. The home test kit does cost £50 and I'm sure the NHS wouldn't put babies lives at risk…

Still, the appointment wasn't all doom and gloom; I got to hear baby's heartbeat - still going good and strong - and my blood pressure and urine test results were all looking good.

In addition, Carol, the midwife, informed me that I was having Braxton Hix contractions. I couldn't feel anything, but she placed my hand on my bump so I could feel where it was hardening. I'd like to think it will be this painless when labour starts for real, but somehow I don't think these so-called 'practise contractions' will really help prepare me. Do you?

April 22 – Week 32

Before I became pregnant I was adamant I would give birth by caesarean. I would insist upon it. I had a number of reasons why. After hearing a selection of horror stories, I'd become convinced that my hips were too small and that my baby would have to be wrenched out of me with forceps – this was exactly what happened to my friend Anna with her first and she's still traumatised 12 year's later.

I was worried about being mutilated down below and left unable to sit down for weeks. I didn't want to become one of the women on the TENA Lady adverts leaking wee every time I laughed or sneezed – which seems to already happened, regardless!

I was eagerly awaiting proposed revisions to the NICE clinical guidelines giving women the right to request a C-Section, but interestingly, when they came I found I had changed my mind.

It was the first visit to the hospital that did it. I know this sounds ridiculous – it is a hospital, after all – but it was so clinical. I hated the size of the place, the smell, the crowds of people and the distinct impression of being on a conveyer belt. That was when I first started thinking about having a home birth. Then, when we spoke to Emily and Simon about their very positive home birth experience, I was sold.

Although not everyone agrees with me, it offers so many benefits. Ultimately, by staying on your home turf you remain in control. The midwives come to you – far preferable than the stress of a car journey and trying to find a space in the over-priced hospital car parks. They stay with you, focusing on you only, rather than any other number of labouring women. You are surrounded by your home comforts – bed, TV, food, bathroom – and, crucially, benefit from the privacy of your own home. Your partner (and whoever else you want) can stay with you throughout without having to wait in a corridor for hours on end. All in all, the whole experience seems far more appealing.

Of course, there are downsides. Namely, the sacrifice of decent pain relief; no one is more surprised than me that I'm choosing an option that offers nothing more than gas and air. But after facing my fears to endure three blood tests since becoming pregnant it's really helped me handle those situations. Add to that the breathing and visualisation techniques taught to us at yoga, and I'm starting to believe I can birth my baby without medical intervention.

Still, it would seem I'm in the minority – I'm the only woman opting for a home birth out of my entire NCT class and those I've told of my plans have more often than not sucked the air between their teeth and uttered "oooh, with your first? You're brave". My midwife Carol is supportive of my choice, however, and recommended I attend a meeting of the local home birth group. It's made up of women who have experienced home births, midwives and doulas, and meets monthly.

I went along on Sunday – equipped with some potato skins made by Tom – for an informal lunch meeting. It was very reassuring to hear their success stories – and even their unsuccessful stories. Several of the women had been planning for home births but had to transfer to hospital at the last minute for various reasons. If there's a problem or any concern, the midwife will just call an ambulance to take you in – that you'll get the best medical care is not something to worry about. In fact, recent research conducted in the Netherlands concluded that giving birth at home is as safe as doing so in hospital. It found no difference in death rates of either mothers or babies in 530,000 births.

In 1960, 33 per cent of women gave birth at home, but by the late eighties this fell to a record low of 0.9 per cent. It's been slowly increasing since, but the most recent figures from the Office for National Statistics show that of all births in England and Wales in 2012, just 2.3 per cent took place at home. So either I'm mad or more needs to be done to promote giving birth at home as a viable option. I hope it's the latter!

April 29 - Week 33

Last session, Nicki the NCT teacher had us draw up a chart listing pain relief options during labour. We were then instructed to work our way through them giving a tick or a cross against various criteria, such as 'are there side effects?' or 'is it controllable?'.

The ones with the most ticks at the end would indicate the best choices, she said. I'm not sure I completely agree, because paracetamol came out very near the top and I don't even find that effective for a mild headache. But, what was visually striking was the multitude of crosses next to the 'serious pain relief' options.

I'd always thought of an epidural as a kind of magic medicine providing a perfect pain-free birth, but I'd never considered the bigger picture. There are lots of negatives. Primarily, that you can't feel contractions and you have to be told when to push. This not only slows the whole process down, the chance of intervention with forceps or ventouse is significantly increased. And because you can't feel what's going on down there, you're much more likely to suffer tearing.

Of course, if you can't feel your lower half, you're confined to your hospital bed and can't benefit from the gravity and friction offered by active birth positions. Then there's the post-birth considerations. The administering of an epidural is not an exact science and it can't be timed to wear off the moment the baby is out. Having to wait to get back on your feet can be detrimental to the successful establishment of breastfeeding. Pethidine, an opiate drug that is also administered by injection, is even worse. It crosses the placenta, can depress baby's breathing and, in many cases, only serves to make the mother feel woozy and nauseous. So, that's right out, even though it is something you can apparently have as part of a home birth.

Perhaps, somewhat surprisingly, what emerged as the ultimate pain relief choice was hypnobirthing – the technique that my friends Emily and Simon were raving about after the birth of their baby back in February. According to Nicki, this method of self-hypnosis has resulted in women claiming completely pain-free experiences. Sounds great, right? But she did add the caveat that it won't work for everyone. If you can't see yourself being able to reach a meditative state, then you probably won't find this effective. I imagine I'm one of those people, but I may still buy a DVD to see what it's all about.

We also talked about TENS machines, which are small portable devices which deliver electrical pulses via stick-on electrode pads. The idea is that the pulsating disrupts the pain signals from reaching the brain. I used to have a Slendertone ab-toning belt, which functioned in a similar way. It was never very effective in helping me achieve a washboard stomach but I do recall how it could make me jump out of my skin if I accidentally knocked it up too high! My friend Kate has lent me a TENS unit anyway, so I'll certainly keep it to hand.

Most encouragingly, the powers of good old-fashioned H2O were highly praised – bathing in it, not drinking it, that is. Immersing oneself in hot water of 36-38 degrees regulates hormones, releases endorphins and relaxes the muscles. It not only speeds up labour and eases pain, it also reduces the risk of tearing as it softens the perineum (the bit between the anus and the vagina). However, you must not enter the water before active labour has started as this can actually slow contractions.

I have now ordered a La Bassine inflatable birth pool from eBay and am looking forward to giving it a dry (or should that be wet) run once it arrives. I had to 'splash' out £70 but once we're through with it, I guess it can double up as a posh paddling pool for the little one!

May 5 – Week 34

This week I have written my 'birth plan'. Quite a few people have said to me that theirs went out the window almost immediately due to unforeseen complications, however I still thought it worthwhile to jot down a little wish list.

Before I started, I had a look at some examples online, which ranged from a tick box template to 1,000 word essays. I decided not to go into detail about candles and music and burning essential oils. Although these are all things I'd like to have, I don't think my midwife needs to concern herself with them. Instead, I've stuck to the key issues like pain relief and labour positions. This is what it looks like:

PLAN FOR HOME BIRTH

Birth partners: My husband Tom and my friend Anna

First Stage

Labouring:
• Use exercise ball
• Employ active labour positions
• Use birth pool

Pain management:
• TENS
• Massage and breathing/relaxation techniques
• Gas and air

Monitoring:
• With waterproof Sonicaid so I don't have to get out of the water

Second Stage

Delivery:
• Episiotomy to be avoided if possible
• Immediate skin to skin
• Wait until umbilical cord has stopped pulsating before cutting
• Husband to be offered the chance to cut the cord

Third Stage

• Natural delivery of placenta (please dispose of the placenta)
• Oral Vitamin K, unless baby has suffered trauma
• Assistance to establish breastfeeding

A maternity nanny I met at a dinner party was the first person to tell me about the benefits of delayed umbilical cord clamping, and I went on to do some further research. Waiting the extra few minutes ensures the baby receives an extra 50 to 100ml of nutrient and oxygen rich blood from the placenta. It's less likely that the baby should have a vitamin K deficiency, hence I've requested only the oral drops rather than the more invasive injection.

I have also decided to wait for natural delivery of the placenta (which can take 10 minutes to one hour), rather than have an injection to speed things up. Taking the natural approach reduces the risk of retained placenta and post partum haemorrhage. It does mean there will be more blood loss at the time of birth but there will be less after – I hear it is common to bleed for six weeks after birth and have been advised to invest in the heftiest of pads!

Other negatives associated with the syntometrine injection are the possibility of the cord snapping or pulling out the uterus, plus it can make you feel sick. I'm sure these are all very small risks, but seeing as I'm going au naturale with the labour, I thought I'd go the whole hog.

Before you start to worry though, I've not gone all hippy on you. I have no intentions of throwing a party and serving up the placenta as pâté, nor am I considering the 'Lotus' method of wrapping the placenta in a Tesco carrier bag and waiting until it shrivels up and drops off the baby. I just hope I'm making the right choices to help my baby boy get off to the best start. Watch this space!

May 14 – Week 35

Today is the first day of the rest of my life. That is a dramatic way of saying I have started maternity leave! Well, actually, that's not quite true; I am on regular leave at the moment because I had some holiday that needed to be used up.

Still, I have five weeks (if baby arrives on schedule) all to myself, to do with whatever I please – how exciting! I posted a message to that effect on Facebook and received a flurry of comments telling me to sleep while I still can…talk about rain on my parade!

Anyway, I have no intention of wasting such precious time sleeping; I have a long list of things I want to do, which I never normally have time for.

These include: making a start on the website for my mat-leave business venture, selling unwanted items on eBay, sorting through my digital photos and creating photo books, editing our wedding video, baking cakes and various arts and crafts projects. I've also made lots of plans to see friends and booked an appointment at the hairdressers. (Hmm…reading that back, five months might be more realistic than five weeks, but it's good to be ambitious, right?)

Tom, ever thoughtful, has treated me to a voucher for a pregnancy massage to celebrate my homecoming, and I'm also feeling very spoilt, with numerous gifts from friends and work colleagues. I do realise I need to make the most of these treats, which are likely to be few and far between once my income is reduced to a paltry £135 a week Statutory Maternity Pay (SMP).

I am worried about how we will cope, but Tom is optimistic about bringing in more business so I'm trying not to think about it too much at this stage. At least as someone who is self-employed he has the opportunity to increase his income. I really don't know how families existing on one average wage, plus basic SMP, manage to make ends meet.

That said, I'm not complaining. It's great that women in the UK are entitled to take 39 paid weeks off work (and a further 13 unpaid, if they want). Amazingly, in the States there is no national law mandating paid time off for new mums, and even unpaid leave is limited to 12 weeks. Pretty much every other country in the world offers a better deal than this! At the other end of the scale is the Czech Republic, where mothers (or fathers) can stay at home for up to four years, whilst benefiting from state support and they must be offered at least the same level position when they do return to work.

I don't know what I'll do yet with regards to returning to work, although I'm pretty sure I won't want to go back full time. With childcare costing an average of £60 a day, it hardly seems worth it on my wage, especially given what I'll miss out on in terms of little man's developments. As far as I'm concerned, my baby's first giggle, first words, first steps are something you just can't put a price on.

Hopefully my little business idea will take off enough to provide the necessary supplement to our household income while offering flexible hours. I'd better get cracking with that website!

May 20 – Week 36

I've gone into a nesting frenzy. I'm finding it impossible just to sit down and relax. Even at night my mind is whirring with all the things I need to do and it's keeping me awake. Still, I have been pleasingly productive over the last few days, washing all of the baby's clothes and blankets with non-bio powder, sorting the clothes into sizes and packing my hospital bag 'just in case'. In my hospital bag I have the following:

Pack of big cotton pants
Maternity pads
Breast pads
Disposable nappies

Wipes
Muslins

And once we have finished mopping up the many bodily fluids…

Big nightie for giving birth in
Pair of PJs and flannel dressing gown
Slippers and socks
Makeup, hairbrush, dry hair shampoo
Wash bag
TENS machine
Two babygrows and two vests
Booties, scratch mitts and hat
Blanket

One thing which I have found very confusing is working out what size clothing my boy will need upon entry to the world. I had purchased a selection of items in 'newborn' – seems logical right? But Anna recently told me that 'newborn' fits up to 9lbs. Given the modest size of my bump, and the fact that both Tom and myself are somewhat vertically challenged, I doubt that he will be that big (at least I hope to God he won't).

The next size down is 'tiny baby', generally up to 7lbs and then 'early baby', usually up to 5lbs, while 0-3 months is up to 12lbs. But to make it even more confusing the sizes vary between different brands. I've gone for the scatter gun approach and got a few of each, which will tide us over until we can get to a shop.

We've also had a trial run inflating the birth pool. It was quick and simple with the electric pump, however when we came to do the base, a funny smell started coming from the pump.

"Do you think there should be a flame inside?" Tom asked.

…umm no. So a good job we did a test run then!

We did have a giggle at the big warning printed on the bottom of the pool: 'strictly no diving!'

"Well, at least it doesn't say no heavy petty," I joked.

As far as mental preparation goes, I received the 'Effective home birth preparation with Maggie Howell' hypnobirthing CD, which I ordered from Amazon and decided to have a listen in the car while driving to see my friend Juliette. When it told me to "close my eyes" I realised it probably was not the best place to do it, but I did some of the visualisation and journeyed in my mind to my favourite beach in Thailand, which did leave me with a feeling of wellbeing.

All in all, I think we're as ready as we can be for little man if he does decide to make an early appearance. If not, I have four more weeks to feather my nest.

May 25 – Week 37

So, the sun has finally come out…and so has another luminous spherical object – my stomach! I was having a proper pregnant lady meltdown yesterday because literally none of my summery clothing would fit; even the stretchy stuff. We're talking t-shirts that would only reach my navel, and skirts that would have exposed the baby's head if I'd bent over.

"I look like Vicky Pollard!" I wailed at Tom, who seemed quite amused by my distress.

"Okay, okay, let's take a trip to Primark and I'll buy you a few bits," he placated.

I would have preferred Seraphine, naturally, but there seems little point in spending lots of money on clothes in my final three weeks. So off we traipsed to 'Primani'; me in my least offensive, but highly unflattering, outfit of brown leggings and a vest top.

I can't say it was an enjoyable experience, pulling on shorts and dresses three sizes larger than normal to see if they would accommodate the bump without making me look deformed, but I did manage to pick up a good selection of basics for under £30. Even Tom couldn't grumble at that.

When I got home I decided to take the scissors to my maternity bootleg jeans and black trousers and make them into pedal pushers. This has proved to be a masterstroke, unless the temperatures take a dramatic plunge back downwards, and then it will be back to Primark!

I thought I'd been so clever making it through my entire pregnancy on just two items of maternity wear but annoyingly these final weeks, which have seen baby (and me) piling on the pounds (babies gain half a pound a week in the last month of pregnancy, apparently), have beaten me.

Perhaps there should be some sort of national maternity clothes recycling scheme with aid packages sent out to desperate women? Or maybe Primark should just pull its finger out and launch a maternity range – how popular would that be?

Anyway, I know how I'm going to treat myself once this baby is out – with a fab pair of coloured skinny jeans!

May 31 - Week 38

Today, children, we're going to talk about vaginas!

I admit that the concept of getting a baby's head out of mine fills me with dread. I'd like to say it's akin to passing a bowling ball through the eye of a needle, but I think Tom would tell me not to flatter myself…

I have had a quiet word with Mother Nature encouraging a design rethink; a Mark 2 fanny for the New Millennium, perhaps with a quick release button, but between you and me, she's a bit of a Luddite.

However, according to my yoga teacher Nadia, perineal massage can be used to pre-stretch 'down below' and make it all a bit easier. She told us that she had tried it herself and successfully given birth without tearing. I decided to ask her for some more information.

The email she sent me was very detailed. Here's an overview:

- Insert two fingers up to the first knuckle into your vagina. Feel what happens when you inhale and exhale
- Place your fingers against the back wall of the vagina – the part nearest to the coccyx. Bring your awareness to this area fully. Breathe deeply until you feel the muscles relax under your fingers on an exhalation
- Repeat this process on the sides of vagina – 10 o'clock and 2 o'clock
- Once you are comfortable with this, continue to the second knuckle so that the stretch becomes deeper

I was a little perturbed by this and let the email languish in my inbox for a few weeks, but with baby due in just two weeks, I decided to be brave and revisit it. I did a bit of further research and found a useful video on YouTube, which demonstrated the process on a model (a plastic one, not a live one!).

So, armed with a ramekin of olive oil, I took myself off to the bathroom to get stuck in, if you'll pardon the pun. The hardest part about it was actually reaching around my bump to get to the area in question. Suggested positions include a leg up on the bath or crouching against a wall, but neither were particularly comfortable, so I gave up pretty quickly. Another suggestion was getting your partner to help, but Tom didn't seem that enthusiastic for some reason!

He did help me with shaving my bush recently. Admittedly it had become a little neglected – well, it's hard to trim when you can't see what you're doing! In the end, I just decided to do away with all the hair as it's easier to maintain myself, and gives the midwife a clear view, I figure.

Speaking of hair, I heard an interesting theory yesterday, which purports that women who suffer bad heartburn will have babies with more hair. It was thought to be a myth, but recent research has shown there to be a correlation. Given my rapacious Gaviscon consumption, it looks like we can expect a yeti!

June 7 – Week 39

So here we are, my baby is due one week today – how exciting! I'm trying not to get too fixated on the date, since only 5 per cent of babies are born on the day they're due, but I have been taking what steps I can to ensure he's not tardy.

These have included regular 'rocking and rolling' sessions on my exercise ball, walking, climbing the stairs and drinking raspberry leaf tea; said to strengthen the uterus. 'Sexy time' has somewhat fallen by the wayside – I don't think either of us have been feeling particularly in the mood, but maybe we'll try to rectify that tonight. I'm guessing I won't want Tom anywhere near that vicinity for some time after birth, so best get some in now.

Anyway, tomorrow I will see the midwife and find out if baby's head is engaged. I'm hopeful it is, since I've had some period cramp sensations low in my pelvis over the last few days, which I've not experienced before.

According to the woman who runs the post office over the road, I'm going to have the baby on Sunday, so that's good. Also, she reckons he's only going to weigh 6lbs, which should make for a relatively easy labour. At the other end of the spectrum, my friend Juliette predicted he would weigh in at a healthy six stone!!

"Six stone? Bloody hell!" I spluttered.

"I meant pounds, six pounds!" she reassured me, although she did add that she thinks the gender scan was wrong, and the baby will in fact be a girl!

That certainly would be a surprise, but not the first Juliette's given me – I arrived home this week to find she'd thrown me a baby shower. My kitchen was full of friends, balloons, bubbly, cakes and presents. I'd written off a baby shower as 'too American', but I've got to admit it was wonderful and I was hugely touched by the effort everyone had gone to. Juliette had even organised for a manicurist to come along to give us all a pamper.

Meanwhile, Elle, who is a photographer, presented me with some fabulous arty studio pictures she'd taken of me, Tom and the bump. There's one where Tom and I have our hands over my bump, forming the shape of a heart, and another where he is kissing my tummy. I really liked it and uploaded it to Facebook as a profile picture. But I didn't leave it there for long. My Mum and Dad rang up to say they'd seen it and thought he was in fact kissing my bum! I wonder how many other people thought that…mortifying!

June 15 – Week 40

So my due date came and went yesterday with not even a twinge in the womb region. I think the most frustrating thing about this wait is the constant barrage of calls, texts and Facebook messages asking me if I've had the baby yet. Trust me folks, when I do, you'll know about it.

I continue to do all the labour-inducing things everyone tells you to do, but like Carol, the midwife, said today:

"The baby won't come until he's ready to come."

Apparently, he is perfectly poised to make his exit but there's just no telling when that might be.

"It could be tonight, it could be in a week," she said.

However, if there's still no sign of him in a couple of days I will go for a membrane sweep, at which point the midwife will also feel my cervix to see if it is softening as it should be.

She did suggest that we might want to engage in some rumpy pumpy (she didn't call it that, obviously, she's a medical professional), which stimulates oxytocin, a hormone which causes contractions. Semen, she added, contains prostaglandin, which is the substance they use to induce birth, inserting it into the vagina as a pessary or gel.

We were told about this at antenatal classes, but Nicki, the teacher, said that it was ten times more effective if the semen was taken orally! Clearly, the husbands had slipped her some cash before the start of the class.

Nicki, however, was adamant that we should not get distressed if our babies were late, stating that in low risk births it was fine for them to stay in utero up to 43 weeks. I've got to say at 40w+1 that's not something I really want to be considering – there just ain't room for the both of us in this body anymore!

She added that in France a full-term pregnancy is considered to be 41 weeks, rather than the 40 weeks calculation we use in the UK. She also said that gestational length often runs in families, so I asked my mum whether she was on time with her first baby. Mum confirmed she was a week late with my older brother and also that her waters didn't break with any of the children except me (I'm one of four). So perhaps this is something to go by?

I have been told that I will be booked for an induction at the hospital at 12 days overdue. Nicki had seemed very negative about inductions, telling us that we could request 'expectant monitoring' instead, as well as a darkened room at the hospital for 'nipple stimulation'!

Sometime later when Tom and I were discussing this with a friend, I discovered that Tom thought the hospital would also provide someone to do it and that it was for sexual pleasure.

"What a great job!" he'd exclaimed.

If I do have to be induced it will ruin my plans for a home birth, but Carol reassured me that I would still be able to go for a water birth at the hospital, which has made me feel a lot more positive about the situation, should it come to that.

For now, it's another night wondering if I'll be woken up by contractions or just the usual need to pee.

THE BIG ARRIVAL

June 21

Welcome to the world baby Archie!

Yes, he finally arrived; exactly one week late, at 16.11 on Thursday June 21 – the Summer solstice. This is how it happened…

The week started with mine and Tom's one-year wedding anniversary. I got some down below action, but sadly not *that* kind; I visited the clinic for a membrane sweep. My cervix was inspected, found to be one centimetre dilated and declared 'favourable'.

Despite the encouraging verdict, nothing happened until Wednesday morning, when I stood up and felt something unusual. It turned out to be my mucus plug coming away (looks like egg whites, sorry if that's too much information). I felt generally 'off' that day (a bit nauseous and tired) and took to bed for a while in the afternoon.

"I think we have a baby on the way," said Tom when he saw me, and sure enough, I was woken at 3.30am the following morning with cramps coming every ten minutes.

We'd been told we weren't supposed to call the midwives until the contractions were five minutes apart so I decided not to wake Tom until 6am. When I did, we lay in bed together and timed the contractions with a special app I'd downloaded on my iPhone. Tom laughed when he noticed it was serving ads for booking.com.

"Talk about inappropriate!" he said.

I can't say I was particularly focused on booking a hotel at the time…

What I wanted to do was get washed and dressed and put on my makeup. I know it seems silly, but I wanted to look nice for such a big occasion. Little did I know how bedraggled I would be in just a few hours!

Anyway, as part of my getting ready, I put on my wedding and engagement rings. I soon realised that was a mistake because my finger started to turn purple. I ran downstairs to Tom shouting "I'm swelling up, help me get these rings off!" and he slathered my hand with the butter he had been spreading on his toast!

At 9am Anna, who I'd asked to be my birth partner, arrived. As my contractions had slowed, we were able to spend the morning chatting, watching TV and eating sweets, while Tom went on a conference call.

"Ooh I think I might have just weed myself a bit," I remarked, alarmed at the warm trickle running down my leg.

"No, you idiot, that'll be your waters", she laughed. Then the next minute she was screaming – one of our cats had run in with a live mouse in his mouth. Anna is petrified of rodents, so I had to get up and chase the cat out – mid contraction!

Around 1pm I had an almighty contraction and actually heard my remaining waters pop. Soon the contractions were coming thick and fast and lasting more than a minute. To add to the discomfort, the contractions were causing my acid reflux to flare up. Every surge sent a wave of burning acid into my throat.

"Gaviscon…" I managed to croak to Tom between contractions. "What's that? You want some Haribo?" he replied, offering me the pack of jelly sweets in his hand.

When I could talk again I told Tom exactly what he could do with his Haribo and he realised it was time to get on the phone to the hospital.

Once the midwife was on her way, he then got down to the all-important business of filling the pool, which was situated in our living room. Unfortunately, we had only tested the hose with cold water and once the boiling hot was going through, the hose expanded and would not stay on the tap. Poor Tom had to hold it in place with a towel as it scalded his hands. Starting to panic, he called our next-door neighbour, Mike, who was luckily working on a job locally. Mike saved the day by running down to Homebase to pick up a different tap connector, but the comedy of errors continued as the man from Green Thumb, the lawn treatment company, appeared in the garden. Thank goodness we had thought to put up some makeshift curtains!

I was *really* starting to need some pain relief by this point, and the midwife had still not arrived. By the time she did, I was collapsed on a yoga mat on the floor, grabbing on to a salad bowl trying not to vomit up the Mars Bar I'd been nibbling on earlier.

The midwife, Mandy, examined me, but I was only five centimetres dilated. She then asked me to get up and go to the bathroom to wee in a receptacle – our kitchen measuring jug! Anna helped me into the loo, propping me up with her shoulder and then helped me off with my dress, as I was getting very hot. I came back through the kitchen in nothing but a red bikini top – It's funny how all dignity goes out the window!

Mandy finally gave me the mouthpiece for the gas and air and I inhaled deeply and gratefully. The sensation was very similar to one I'd experienced at a music festival a few years ago after taking a pill of the non-prescription variety. While I could still feel the pain, I was somewhat removed from the situation and was able to cope.

Eventually, I was able to get into the pool, at around 2.30pm. Submersing myself in the hot water was a huge relief but I was still fiercely sucking on the gas and air. I started to panic when I heard Mandy on the phone asking for a second canister to be brought because we were about to run out.

"I can't be without it," I told Anna desperately.

Thankfully, a second canister arrived quickly, along with my regular midwife Carol – and an involuntary urge to start pushing. It came in waves, which climaxed with a big push and a loud, primal scream (my poor neighbours!). It was kind of like upside down retching – my body just took over.

Tom had the unenviable job of maintaining the pool temperature at exactly 37 degrees and was running back and forth with hot water from the stove and cold water from the kitchen tap. He tells me he felt like someone trying to put out a fire in the medieval ages!

Although for most of the labour I was completely zoned out, I did have one or two moments of clarity. Once when I became aware of the ridiculous yellow digital duck thermometer bobbing past me in the water and again when I noticed a small poo floating in the water. I pointed at it and said 'poo' in a pathetic voice. No friend or lover should have to see that, but they were both very discreet about it!

Everybody kept telling me I was doing well and making good progress, but I was convinced they were lying to me and kept thinking 'why didn't I just go to the hospital and have an epidural?'. Just when I thought I could go on no longer, my body convulsed and with a giant push I felt the head come out.

"One more push" they said and his body slipped easily out into the water.

"He's here," they said. "Pick him up!"

I was completely in shock and took a few seconds to register, before reaching down into the water and scooping him up into my arms. I stared at his tiny face, taking in every detail – he was perfect! He was pink and slippery and had a head of light brown hair. I just couldn't get over the fact he had come out of me.

I held him close while the placenta finished pulsating and then Tom was handed the scissors to cut the cord. The water in the pool had turned crimson and the midwives were worried about blood loss. They asked if I would have the injection to speed up delivery of the placenta, which would allow them to inspect me for tearing. I quickly agreed – the cord was hanging from between my legs and I just wanted it out as soon as possible. Once the injection had been administered, it plopped out pretty much instantly and, starting to feel somewhat woozy, I decided to avert my eyes.

The good news was that the tearing was minimal – about an inch – and Carol appropriated the anglepoise lamp from the office to light the way as she stitched me up. Ironically, being injected with anaesthetic in my sore and battered nether regions was one of the most acutely painful parts! Anna – again going above and beyond the call of duty – cleaned the blood off my legs and helped me back to the loo, where I was advised to apply not one giant maternity pad, but two!

Archie, as we named him, was weighed and inspected (coming in at 7lbs on the nose) and then dressed by Anna before finally being placed back in my arms. My work was over, but for hardworking Tom 'Operation Clean Up' had only just begun!

"So how am I supposed to get the water out?" he asked.

I told him I was sure the pool came with a submersible pump but he couldn't find it anywhere and I was in no state to help him look.

"We'll just have to do it the hard way then – bucket by bucket."

Trust me when I say there was a LOT of water in the pool, and full of all sorts of unmentionables. The poor guy spent the next hour and a half running back and forth to the garden. The flowerbed now looks like something out of 'The Day of the Triffids'.

Eventually, two very tired, but completely elated new parents were able to sit back and just gaze at their beautiful newborn son.

"We made this," we said proudly. "Aren't we clever!"

EARLY DAYS

June 29 – 1 Week

My first week of being a mother has been both challenging and wonderful in equal measures. One thing I had not anticipated is that breastfeeding would be so hard. It is supposed to be 'the most natural thing in the world', so who knew it would not come naturally?

Archie mustn't have been paying attention during the latching-on lesson at baby school because he just didn't seem to know what to do. Everything I read in books and all the tutorials I watched on YouTube advised that putting the baby 'nose to nipple' would result in a nice wide gape, and baby getting a big mouthful of boob. In practice, he would just have a little lick and within a few minutes be fast asleep.

The midwife who visited me the day after the birth told me to try expressing my colostrum, but all I could manage were a few measly drops – not nearly enough to satisfy him. And come 2am the following morning he was wailing with hunger. It's the most heartbreaking sound I've ever heard.

And so, bleary eyed and desperate, Tom and I headed down to the kitchen to fix him up a bottle of ready-made Aptamil (I'd bought a few cartons on the advice of a friend). We gave him 70ml and he drank greedily. We offered him some more at 6am, which was also consumed with gusto. But when my midwife Carol visited later that morning, we were told off for giving him such large quantities – his stomach is only the size of a two pence coin, we were told – and by giving him a bottle, we had jeopardised establishing breastfeeding.

I felt terrible, and with each failed attempt to get Archie to latch, a little more of my confidence eroded. It didn't help that we had a house full of relatives – my parents, Tom's mum and Rosie were all staying with us and each time I wanted to try him on the breast I had to leave the room for privacy. If we were to make this work, I knew what we really needed was some peace and quiet and lots of skin-to-skin time. I also felt in need of more support from Tom – he was spending so much time looking after our visitors and being a good host that in my exhausted and emotional state I felt I was doing it all alone.

When Tom asked me how I was doing I broke down in tears.

"I don't think I can do this," I told him.

He reassured me, said we would clear the house of visitors and encouraged me to hang on until the next day's midwife visit. That visit, from Mandy, was a lifesaver.

She started by telling me that if I wanted to switch to formula, then I could. No one would judge me and it wouldn't do the baby any harm. It was the first time a medical professional had presented that as an option and it was such a relief to hear. I asked her what would have happened in the old days, before formula, if a baby wouldn't feed and she said simply that they would have 'failed to thrive' i.e. died.

She pointed out that my breasts were engorged and must be sore, and showed me how to massage them. She helped me get going on the breast pump and we devised a plan to express every three hours. I could feed Archie this in the bottle and top him up with formula, if required.

Having a positive course of action felt great although getting up at all hours and sticking a noisy milking machine to my nipples wasn't a fantastic experience. Because my breasts were round and hard with milk, I couldn't get it to attach properly (not even the breast pump will latch on!!) and fumbling around with it in my zombie-like state at 2am was enough to bring me to tears. However, after Googling the problem, I found a solution by removing the rubber cover and putting the plastic cup directly to my boob.

The sensation is rather unpleasant and my poor nipples look grossly misshapen afterwards, but at least I can harvest a decent amount this way. Despite the success with the expressing, I had not given up completely on returning Archie to the boob. Another midwife advised that I try a nipple shield – a thin piece of perforated rubber, which covers the nipple. The idea was that he would be fooled into thinking it was a bottle and give it a good suck. He did show a bit more interest, but my nipples were too small to fill them and it was basically a fiddly, slippery mess.

By the time another midwife called in on day five, I had pretty much resigned myself to the fact that Archie was not a boob man and that I would express for just a few more days before swapping to formula. But this midwife was of the 'breast is best' brigade and encouraged me to attend a breastfeeding clinic at the hospital the following day.

I didn't think I would bother, but the next day I decided giving it one last shot would allow me to change to bottle-feeding with as little guilt as possible. I was greeted at the breastfeeding clinic by a *very* old lady. She had a hairy upper lip, smelt of cheese and onion and was clutching a knitted boob - I was not inspired with confidence.

She told me to strip Archie off, take my bra off and lay him across my chest. She chuckled and cooed over him and said "what a bonny baby!" but thankfully a midwife from the younger generation was also on hand. She tried him in the underarm position, lined him up just so and, what do you know, he latched on and started guzzling! He fed for 20 minutes before falling off into a deep contented sleep.

We have managed to continue successfully at home over the last couple of days, allowing me to abandon the dreadful twilight pumping and instead pull Archie into bed with me, although we have maintained a 2am bottle feed of expressed milk, enabling Tom to do his bit and me to get some unbroken sleep. I am so pleased Archie has finally got the hang of it, although I am still quite the rooky when it comes to mothering.

Tom and I ventured out for our first family day trip today, to the spa town of Tunbridge Wells. We decided to just carry Archie in the sling and not bother with the pushchair to make wandering the cobbled lanes easier. However this unfortunately meant there was nowhere to put him when we sat down in a restaurant for lunch. Later, as we were stood looking in a shop window, I felt a warm liquid dribbling on my foot. Archie's nappy was leaking and he was wet through, but silly Mummy had not thought to bring a change of clothes. So off we went to Boots to buy a pack of bodysuits - as well as a changing bag, so we can carry all those baby necessities about our person. Travelling light has become a thing of the past I think.

We did buy one other thing today – Archie's first shoes. A teeny tiny pair of Converse Hi-Tops, in red, just like Mummy's. I'm not one for dressing my baby in a load of designer gear (they only puke and crap all over it) and I know he won't really need to wear shoes for many months, but these were just too cute to resist.

All in all it was a lovely day and hopefully the first of many this summer has in store.

July 5 – 2 Weeks

Archie has been feeding brilliantly; he is gaining weight and seems as happy as a sand boy. So, all should be rosy, right? Except what's really rosy is the colour of my nipples, which have taken quite a battering and are now covered in little blisters. Archie has turned into quite the champion sucker and now seems to want to feed every two hours, whereas before it was only every three – and we were often having to wake him for them. His appetite is insatiable. He'll guzzle at a nipple for 40 minutes, have a sleep for ten minutes and then want to get back on. Frankly, it's painful, exhausting and I don't think I can take much more of it. It's getting to the point where I'm dreading feeding Archie. This is not the picture perfect vision of mother and baby bonding described at antenatal class.

I'm so disappointed with myself. After all the bother getting him to feed, and being so pleased when we succeeded, I'm now back at square one, wondering how soon I can switch to formula without hating myself for being a bad mum?

In addition to my sore boobs, I've been suffering with chronic constipation. Every time I want to go I have to spend half an hour trying to pass grotesquely large, dry stools, ripping my bottom in the process. Honestly, it's like giving birth again – but without the gas and air! I have been advised to take Lactulose sugar syrup by the pharmacist, which is one of the few laxatives that is safe to use while breastfeeding (and tastes pretty good too). Hopefully that will get things moving again.

Archie has also had a touch of constipation. As promised, he successfully delivered us the black tarry meconium explosion, and then some delightful 'korma poo', but after that, nothing. We weren't too worried at first, having read that breastfed babies may not go that often, but after five days of nothing but wet nappies, we were getting a little concerned. A midwife came out to check Archie over. She felt his stomach to see if there was a blockage, but found it to be nice and soft. She showed me how to 'cycle' his legs and massage his tummy to help things along, and said if nothing had happened within 24 hours, we could give him half an ounce of freshly squeezed orange juice mixed with half an ounce of boiling water.

We happened to have an orange in the fruit bowl, so I mixed the concoction up for him that evening…and hey presto, by 5am we had a poo! I'd never been so delighted to see one before. Still, they say you should be careful what you wish for; it now seems like every nappy is a dirty one (and he's farting like a trooper too) …

While we're on the topic of bodily functions; Sylvester, one of our cats, has started pissing everywhere. He is clearly most put out by the new arrival and decided to make this known by blatantly weeing on Archie's play mat – all while Tom was watching and shouting at him. Naturally upset with him, we gave him the cold shoulder that evening, further compounding his displeasure, and when I came to take Archie out in his (brand new) car seat the next day, I found a big smelly cat piss in it. This meant I couldn't take Archie out, so I was not pleased at all, as you can imagine.

I popped in to see the vet to ask if there was anything I could do to prevent the pee protest. She told me about a product called Feliway; a synthetic pheromone, which can be pumped out by a room diffuser and makes the cat think it has already marked all of its territory. We haven't got our hands on any yet, but Tom and I have been making an effort not to ignore the cat.

To be fair I can understand his indignation, we did dote on him as our furry baby until this hairless thing that does nothing but cry turned up and usurped him. We hope a bit of extra attention will reassure Sylvester of his position in the household but Tom's mum isn't taking any risks; she's already been out and bought us a cat net for Archie's Moses basket just in case he gets it in his head to smother him!

July 12 – 3 Weeks

I'm sorry to report that the battle of the breast is over. After a little over two weeks I made the very difficult decision to switch exclusively to formula. Pretty pathetic, I know, but between breastfeeding, expressing and topping up with formula, I was both mentally and physically exhausted. At least Archie is in rude health. The midwife who came to weigh him in order to discharge him had to check the scales.

"Ooh that seems like a lot in a few days," she said, lifting him off and setting him back down. "Nope, that's right," she confirmed. "He's obviously feeding well!"

It appears he had regained his birth weight and added an additional eight ounces.

I asked her about the best way to stop breastfeeding to minimise the risk of mastitis – I had read numerous advice online, from winding down slowly to going cold turkey. She advised the latter, taking paracetamol for the discomfort or hand expressing a little in the bath if very engorged. So I stopped on Sunday and waited with trepidation for the arrival of breasts of stone. It didn't take long. By that evening I was already considering giving the baby a sneaky go on them, but the midwife had said that would only continue to stimulate them, and I had to be clear about my decision. Hormonally, it was tough not to respond to my baby's cry in the way nature intended. At one point I lifted my bra away to have a look at my nipple and a drop of milk instantly materialised. It appeared to me as a teardrop my breast was crying because I wouldn't let it do its job – I told you I was hormonal.

However, it's now Thursday and my breasts have returned to their normal soft and squidgy texture, the leakages have gone and my nipples – although a little crusty – are no longer sore.

Now I'm out the other side, with a three/four hourly feeding schedule established and my sanity restored, I feel happy with the decision. That's not to say I don't feel some guilt and a little disappointed with myself that I couldn't stick it out, but overall I think it's better for me and, therefore, better for Archie.

I'm revelling in the freedom of being able to leave the house without having to worry about where we'll be at feeding time and it means I can select whatever I like to wear, without having to think about booby access. It also means other people can enjoy feeding Archie – and have been.

We've had scores of adoring visitors, laden with gifts, in the last few weeks. In fact, I have written and sent nearly 50 thank you cards (now there's something I wouldn't have had time to do if I was still breastfeeding!).

We've had some lovely presents, although there does seem to have been a definite theme, with six summer dungaree outfits. Sadly, I think it will be winter before he's in them, because despite gaining weight rapidly, he's still a tiddler and just grown into 'newborn' size.

Not that we've had much of a summer so far. Besides the one sunny day when we went to Tunbridge Wells, it's been rain, rain, rain. Archie and I have been getting together with the NCT girls and their babies for regular buggy walks but we've been having to go armed with umbrellas, wellies, waterproof coats and rain covers.

Archie doesn't seem to mind the water though, and is loving his baths now that his umbilical cord stump has fallen off and he can be fully submerged. I made bath time even more of a treat last night, by finishing off with a massage. I used some Bio Oil and gently massaged it in, starting with his feet and making my way up to his shoulders. He seemed very relaxed afterwards and we had a nice peaceful night. Now, if only I can persuade Tom to give it a go on me…

ONE MONTH OLD

July 19 – 4 Weeks

From one extreme to the other; Archie's constipation last week has transitioned to constant diarrhoea. Typically, it started on the day I decided to start him on cloth nappies. After the delivery of two foul packages, I decided to temporarily go back to the Pampers.

I'd hoped it would clear up overnight, but it was still going strong in the morning. As a fretful first time mum I'd started to worry, but I was due to take him to be weighed, so I was able to consult the health visitor. She said to wait another 24 hours and if he was still suffering, to make an appointment with his GP.

The runs did indeed remain, but as it was Sunday and the surgery was closed, we had to call the out of hours service. Although Archie didn't have a temperature and was still feeding well, they agreed we should see a doctor, just to be on the safe side. We made the appointment for 4pm, as we were due at Pizza Express for an NCT reunion lunch, now the last of the babies has been born. But no sooner had we put down the phone, than little Archie threw up his entire last feed. Now I was really worried, so we rescheduled and got ourselves straight down to the hospital.

Fortunately, after checking him over, the doctor wasn't too concerned. She said that as long as he continued to eat at least half of his usual feeds he shouldn't be at risk of dehydration. She recommended feeding little and often, offering a small amount of boiled water in between if his lips looked dry and lathering plenty of barrier cream on his sore little bottom.

As for the cause, she said it was probably a virus and asked if Tom or I had had upset tummies. We both realised we had, but what amounted to some unusual gurgles for us, naturally had far more of an impact on him. In fact, we are now on day seven of loose bowel movements, but thankfully, the frequency has significantly decreased to two in 24 hours, instead of every nappy change.

Otherwise, he seems very well; getting heavier every day (he's tracking the 25th centile nicely) and practising his smiling – I'm sure we're going to get a proper, unmistakable smile any day now. I am somewhat distressed, however, that he is losing his lovely head of hair. He seems to be cultivating a monastic tonsure; bald on top and long on the sides. It was so long at the back, it was starting to look like a mini mullet. Apparently it is a hairstyle that babies on my husband's side of the family tend to sport (including him and Rosie). I said to Tom that we either embrace the look and give Archie an earring and a neckerchief, or I take the scissors to it – we decided on the latter.

I'm sure Archie would thank me for it if he could. I've been studying baby body language (according to 'The Baby Whisperer' Tracy Hogg) and feel I'm actually starting to understand him quite well. It's just a matter of deduction really; if I know he's not hungry or needing a nappy change, than it can only be wind or tiredness or perhaps needing a cuddle. We're blessed that he has a very amenable nature and only seems to cry if one of his above needs has not been met – what Tracy Hogg calls an 'Angel Baby'.

To be honest, I think Archie's just pretty lazy. When he's not feeding, he spends most of the time asleep (about 17 hours a day!). I'm by no means complaining about his slumbering, but the short periods of quiet alertness he does have are just so wonderful. He studies my face with those beautiful blue eyes and grasps my finger with his tiny hand. My heart just swells with love for the little fella. I think it will simply explode the first time he calls me Mummy!

July 26 – 5 Weeks

At a recent NCT coffee morning the conversation turned to sex (as it often does when a group of girls get together). One of the mums wanted to know how many of us had got back in the saddle, so to speak. Although she was the first among us to have her baby back in in early April, she confessed that she had not yet been intimate with her husband because she was suffering from bladder weakness and was worried about having an accident.

Another girl, who had been nervous about doing it again, said she had been advised by her doctor to 'use plenty of KY Jelly and just do it', while another mum had dabbled with some foreplay but not yet gone all the way.

I have been studiously avoiding my nether regions, waiting for it all to shrink back into place and to get the A-Okay at my six-week check, but, after our conversation, I decided to be brave and let Tom take a look.

I was concerned about what he would see – a gaping black hole, with unidentified fleshy bits hanging down? I was also concerned about what he would feel – would it be like throwing the proverbial hot dog down a hall way? I waited with trepidation while he delivered his verdict.

"It looks a bit different," he declared.

"Different in what way?"

"Well, the opening looks a bit bigger."

I've got to say, this didn't make me feel particularly sexy, but Tom seemed very keen so I agreed to some further exploration, providing he took it very slowly.

He did, and it was actually fine; quite enjoyable, in fact. It didn't feel any different to me, and he said it didn't feel any different to him either. It was nice to get back to the missionary position, which had been an impossibility for so many months because of the front bumper.

Something else I did this week that I've not done in a long time was have a proper night out. I wouldn't necessarily have chosen to leave Archie for an entire evening at just five weeks, but it was to celebrate two close friends' birthdays and I couldn't let them down.

It felt odd getting glammed up, stepping into a little dress and high heels and kissing my little boy goodbye, but my mum was staying down with us and was clearly pleased to be helping look after him.

As we stood in the crowded bar, with music pumping, I had to fight away the thought that I shouldn't be there. A few drinks helped me relax, but I kept my phone out in case it rang and touched in with a text to Tom a couple of hours later.

"He's been smiling!" he said, when I asked how baby was.

"Proper smiles? Noooo he can't do that when I'm not there!" I replied.

Then he sent me a picture (pretty mean, eh?). He was kind of smiling, but I bet it had taken Tom about 10 minutes to capture it on camera. Still, it made me miss him lots, and I showed it proudly to all my friends and the random guys who were attempting to chat us up. For the record, it didn't seem to deter them that I was happily married and had just had a baby!

I did leave the party early, but it was a good tonic to let my hair down and hang out with the girls. And when I gave baby boy his night-time feed I found he had saved a smile for me. Pure magic.

August 2 – 6 Weeks

While there are benefits to formula feeding, one of the distinct disadvantages is the cost. Archie is currently chomping his way through a £10 tub a week, and will soon be getting through two of them (there goes the Child Benefit money I had been planning to spend on cigarettes and alcohol).

In an effort to economise, I looked into the possibility of buying formula in bulk, but was interested to learn that strict government guidelines prevent any discounting or special offers. You can't even collect supermarket loyalty points on it and the manufacturers are forbidden from promoting it.

That explains why I keep getting bizarre emails from SMA and Aptamil about breastfeeding; its benefits, how to do it, what nursing mothers should be eating etc. When I went onto Aptamil's website, looking for information about their products, I actually had to read a notice about breastfeeding before being allowed to continue.

Then I read an article about a hospital in New York, which has placed its formula under lock and key and is requiring midwives to give mothers a lecture on the benefits of breastfeeding before allowing them access.

I do appreciate that 'breast is best' but I don't agree with shoving it down people's throats, if you'll pardon the expression. For mums who were planning to breastfeed, but for whatever reason find they cannot, this policy will do nothing but make them feel inadequate and depressed.

The fact of the matter is, that while more than eight out of 10 mothers in the UK start breastfeeding their babies, just 45 per cent are still doing so by the time their babies are six to eight weeks old (according to a 2011 survey by the NHS Information Centre). Yes, more should be done to support them to continue – if that is what they wish to do – but those who don't should also be supported.

The NCT antenatal classes did a whole session on breastfeeding but failed to cover bottle-feeding completely. As I had planned to express milk, I had purchased bottles and a steriliser in advance and also a few cartons of readymade formula (on the advice of a friend). But another friend, Rachel, had not been so prepared. She told me how her newborn baby (now two) was screaming the house down with hunger at midnight. She wished she could 'top him up' with formula, but she had absolutely no equipment. No one had told her that breastfeeding might not be totally straightforward.

I struggled to find official advice on how to safely make up bottles in advance/what to do if you are going out and won't have access to a kettle. It was another mum who came to my rescue, as I stood in the baby aisle of Tesco complaining to Tom that we couldn't afford to feed Archie exclusively on the readymade cartons.

She explained about filling sterilised bottles with boiled water and storing them until needed, when you could simply add the formula and serve at room temperature. She told me about the little sectioned pots you can get, which hold three portions of formula and advised me on special bottles available for colicky babies. I can't tell you how grateful I was to that lady.

Bottle-feeding using this system has made life so much simpler and straightforward. It's so easy, in fact, that it kind of makes me feel guiltier for not breastfeeding; like I'm not prepared to put any effort in or make any sacrifices for my son (if that makes any sense?). The other mums from antenatal group are all sat there with babies permanently clamped to their boobs, while my baby takes a bottle and then goes to sleep for several hours leaving me free to do whatever I please. Clearly I've opted for easy street and there must be a price to pay for it, right?

When Archie got diarrhoea, it did cross my mind that if he'd been getting the antibodies from my milk then he might not have. I was discussing it with my mum when she revealed: "You were bottle fed from the word go and it didn't do you any harm".

I don't know why, but I'd always presumed I was breastfed. Apparently, after breastfeeding two of my brothers and combination feeding the other, she'd just had enough. This made me feel a lot happier. We'll never know if I would have been healthier/cleverer/happier if I'd been breastfed (I'm sure Freud would have something to say about it), but I don't think I've turned out too badly.

Happily, the doctor seemed delighted with Archie's development at his six-week check. I was a little concerned that he was feeding too much (he's taking four to five ounces every three to four hours) but he said, at 10lbs 1 ounce, he's shaping up as he should be.

"He's perfect," said the doctor, adding: "As you make such lovely babies you'll have to have another."

I thanked him for the compliment but said I'd just take a prescription for the contraceptive pill for the time being…

August 10 – 7 Weeks

Archie slept through to nearly 6am this morning! I'm so proud of him. We really couldn't have asked for a better baby.

We've been giving him a late night 'dream feed' at 11pm for a couple of weeks (as recommended by The Baby Whisperer), but last night was the first time I put him to bed before then. We had been letting him doze in his rocker downstairs during the evening, but I decided that at seven weeks it was probably time to start establishing a proper bedtime. I changed him into his 'PJs' before his 8pm feed and then settled him down in his Moses basket around 9pm. We have a fantastic video monitor so I could sit downstairs and watch the telly but still keep a watchful eye on him.

When the time for his dream feed arrived he was still fast asleep and at first I didn't think he would take his bottle. His mouth hung slack as I tried to tempt him with the teat, but then he started sucking. He finished the whole lot off in his sleep, his eyes tightly shut throughout – I guess that's why they call it the dream feed!

Taking the advice of The Baby Whisperer, I didn't burp him or change his nappy, just settled him straight back down before going to bed myself. I couldn't believe it when I opened my eyes, checked the clock, and saw it was 5.50am.

He was making a few noises but wasn't crying. When I went to his Moses basket he was awake but seemed quite happy. If I can get him to go an hour or two longer, I won't need to go back to bed afterwards, which might mean I can get myself together to leave the house before 11am – always an achievement!

I need to start putting some time aside for exercising; I'd like to commit to a weekly yoga and Zumba class (two separate classes, you understand, not yoga-Zumba, although that could be interesting!). Yesterday I dragged my cross trainer out from behind the shed and – literally – dusted off the cobwebs. I did ten minutes and almost keeled over. I was fortunate not to put on much weight during my pregnancy (quite a feat given my cake consumption), but clearly my fitness has suffered and I do need to tighten up my jelly belly.

My friend Kate said I should get myself along to my nearest Buggyfit session, which basically involves a bunch of women running along with their buggies but I think I might feel like a bit of an idiot.

Still, needs must if I'm to get back into those super skinny jeans. I have two pairs that I bought just before I fell pregnant and consequently have barely worn them. I am back in most of my clothes, however, and took great delight in throwing out my maternity garments.

Meanwhile, I managed to sell my despised breast pump and Dreamgenii pregnancy pillow on eBay and shall be putting the money towards a pedicure and a shopping trip!

August 16 – 8 Weeks

I don't remember much from school, but I do remember learning one thing that made a real impression on me (ok, two things; the condom on the banana sex-ed lesson scarred me for life). We learned that a disposable nappy can take up to 500 years to biodegrade. We also learned that an average baby gets through around 6,000 nappies before being toilet trained.

My young mind boggled at these figures and I wondered why we weren't surrounded by fields and fields of soiled nappies. I made a promise to myself that if I were ever to have kids (although that was highly unlikely because I thought boys were smelly and gross), I would do the 'green' thing and use washable nappies.

When I found out I was pregnant, I started looking into washables and was overwhelmed by the different options. However, having <u>never</u> put any kind of nappy on a child before, what I wanted was the simplest. I chose the TotsBots Easyfit all in one, which has an integral waterproof outer and goes on just like a disposable. They come in fab designs and have a one-size-fits-all popper system. I invested in five of them, but knew this would not be enough.

I then found someone selling a job lot of 15 TotsBots Bamboozle nappies on eBay for £50 and snapped them up. These ones have a separate waterproof cover, but still looked pretty easy to use.

I had already made a deal with myself that I would use disposables for the first month, just until I'd had time to figure out which end of the baby did what. This turned out to be extremely fortunate, since our washing machine broke down the day after I gave birth – sublime timing!

The switch to washables was further delayed, however, by Archie's diarrhoea, which lasted nearly a fortnight, so we've only recently got round to trying them properly. It's not going particularly well.

I'd love to say they were fantastic, but the absorbency does not come anywhere close to that of a Pampers nappy. We've had leak after leak; on his new trousers, on his play mat, on Tom's lap. I've been having to change him every couple of hours because as soon as he's done a wee he becomes uncomfortable. I've also noticed that the wee is absorbed across the whole nappy, so he's wet around his tummy – not very nice.

On a practical level, it is difficult fitting them under his clothes. These days, baby clothes are just not designed with a big cloth butt in mind. Anna was not impressed when she saw Archie in them.

"What are you using these horrible big bulky things for?" she asked.

I tried to explain about the 6,000 nappies and the 500 years but she didn't seem to be listening. She's convinced the washables are going to give Archie some kind of deformity because of the way they push his legs into a wide froggy position.

I told her I wasn't overly worried about this, since generations of babies have worn cloth nappies and gone on to walk successfully, but I had to admit to being disappointed with them (hard when I've spent over £100 on the blooming things).

I think today's leak – all over the nursing chair - is the last straw. Tom declared 'this isn't working' and I had to agree. I guess we've been spoilt by our six weeks of Pampers and all the reliability and convenience they offer. I haven't completely given up my eco crusade however; I'm going to try out some biodegradable disposables, although they are significantly more expensive.

Alternatively, maybe I can just train Archie to use the toilet? Marie from my NCT group says she takes her three-month-old daughter Phoebe to the toilet every morning at 6am and dangles her over the pan while she does a poo!! Another friend of ours has trained her Bengal cat to poo in the loo (although he can't flush, like Jinxy in 'Meet the Fockers'), so it would seem anything is possible!

TWO MONTHS OLD

August 21 – 9 Weeks

Archie, Today you are two months old. I don't know where the time has gone! You are getting so big – you've almost outgrown your Moses basket.

Daddy and I are getting to know you a little bit more with every day that passes. This is what we've learned about you:

You love bath time. You like being soaped up and rinsed off with a stream of water squeezed from a sponge high above your head and tummy.

You have ticklish feet and giggle when we play with them.

You are at your smiliest after a sleep and especially first thing in the morning. You even smile in your sleep and make the cutest squeaks and sighs when you are dreaming. And, when you wake, you have a big stretch, pushing out your chest and pouting your lips.

You think Daddy is for fun and Mummy is for cuddles and often, when I feed you, you stare at me so intently I wonder what you're thinking.

You are a happy little soul and quite content to amuse yourself by smiling at the toys dangling over your chair or the mirror on your play mat.

You don't cry very often, but when you do, it's the sweetest little cry and you are easily comforted by a pat on the back or a stroke on the cheek.

You have the ability to turn your face an alarming shade of beetroot in an instant, returning to a normal colour equally quickly.

You always seem to have fluff in the palms of your balled up little fists and I just don't know where you get it from!

You sleep – a lot. If we take you out, you almost always sleep through the entire outing and then wake up once we get back home. You must wonder why we never go anywhere!

I'm looking at you while I write this and your eyelids are drooping… oops you're asleep.

August 30 – 10 Weeks

I'm a wimp, I admit it. Archie had to have his first vaccinations and I made Tom take him in, while I stayed in the waiting room. I knew it would break my heart to hear him cry and I didn't want him to pick up on my anxiety.

He was quiet and subdued when he came out, except for occasional deep sobs. I'd never heard him like that before and it was somehow even more distressing than out and out wailing. Still, we both got over it and I feel relieved that he is now protected against diphtheria, tetanus, polio and whooping cough, which Tom suffered with when he was tiny and I heard on the news is making a comeback.

I took Archie to visit his grandparents up in Lincolnshire for a few days earlier this week, leaving Tom at home. It was lucky we were travelling alone because there was very little space left in the car once I was finished packing. There was the pushchair, rocker, pop-up Moses basket, bedding, electric steriliser, bottles, tub of formula, bath cradle, towel and toiletries, enough nappies for four days and multiple changes of clothes. Honestly, the preparation was military!

I was a little bit daunted by the prospect of the 150 mile journey because we have a rearward facing car seat, which fits in the back and I knew I wouldn't be able to monitor Archie as closely as I like to. I'd heard there was a risk of babies' heads drooping forward while asleep in car seats, cutting off their breathing and was paranoid about it. I spent the journey continually checking my rear-view mirror for signs of life and always breathed a sigh of relief when I saw a foot twitch. We made a stop two hours in at motorway services, where I changed and fed him before getting back on the road.

We arrived safe and sound and Grandma and Granddad had a great time catching up on cuddles with Archie and cooing about how much he'd grown. It was the first time Archie had been away from his daddy and Tom called that evening to say he was already missing him terribly. He did, however, have a plan to make the most of being home alone – a 'boys behaving badly' night out on the town with friends, followed by a poker night with the NCT dads. He confessed to some 'championship drinking' and was still in a sorry state by the time we got home the next evening.

"Don't worry; I won't be doing it again for while," he promised. "I'm too old for it!"

I was pleased to have successfully made the trip, as a test run for a longer stay away from home – hopefully abroad – which we plan to have in a month or two. We'll certainly have to try and pack a bit lighter, however. A friend told me about a company called Bebebel which delivers your usual brand of nappies, milk, food and other items direct to your holiday resort, which sounds like a great idea.

Archie has already got his first passport. It's a ridiculous document to be honest – the photo was taken at a just few weeks old and shows a scrunched up little face with eyes closed. It already looks nothing like him and it's valid until he is five years old! However, my friend Kate gave us a lovely baby blue leather cover and I'm sure we'll still be the proudest parents going the first time we hand it over at passport control!

September 6 – 11 Weeks

When is a dress not a dress? When it's a Christening gown. At least that's my story and I'm sticking with it. Tom and I had a slight disagreement over Archie's outfit for his baptism this Sunday. I wanted him to wear the Victorian silk gown that I wore and has been in my family for generations, but Tom said he "didn't want his son wearing a dress". I decided to put it out to public vote and posted a picture of Archie in his gown on Facebook.

To be honest, I expected lots of comments about being old fashioned and for Tom to say 'I told you so', but the general consensus was that tradition is good and that Archie looked 'cute'. So I won after all!

The fact that we were having this debate at all was frankly a surprise, as I'd always said I would not have my child baptised. But then I always said I wouldn't get married in a church…

It would seem I'm quite the hypocrite! So what's changed? Not my religious beliefs (or absence of them), but becoming a wife and mother has made me terribly sentimental and eager to cling onto family tradition. I was baptised, and so was my husband, and it somehow seems right that our son should be too.

Tom's mum is actually very religious and it means a lot to her. She's delighted by the opportunity to dig the top tier of our wedding cake out of the freezer, where she's been storing it for this very purpose for the last 14 months.

It's also a great excuse to get all our friends and family together to officially celebrate Archie's arrival. And to be really cynical, it won't harm when it comes to getting him into the best school.

This week we actually visited a nursery to check it out ahead of my return to work next year. The good ones are always over subscribed so you have to get in early!

We're lucky that it's only a few doors down and is rated 'outstanding' by OFSTED. It was lovely; very well run and full of fantastic activities for the children. A member of staff was even playing the guitar and singing Coldplay songs to them! I was surprised at how positive I felt about Archie going there; I had worried I would feel like I was abandoning him but I think he'll really benefit from going there and, crucially, really enjoy it. I've signed him up for two days a week at £48 a day, although I'm yet to have the discussion with work about returning part time or figure out the financials. I'm sure it will all work out and we're not committed to it if our plans change.

I can't believe I'm already four months into my leave. Things are going so quickly. We've even moved Archie into his cot this week, as there was very little space left his Moses basket. Thankfully, the transition didn't seem to bother him at all! We did ease him into it a bit by first moving his Moses basket from our room into his.

As much as I loved having him close, it has meant sounder sleep for Tom and I. He's a noisy little munchkin; squeaking, sighing and thrashing about and I'm attuned to his slightest murmur. Now he's next door we only hear the noises we need to hear.

It did take us a couple of nights to feel relaxed about leaving him alone, with both Tom and I having anxiety dreams. I dreamed about Archie's cot collapsing (perhaps this says more about my faith in Tom's DIY skills?), while Tom dreamed about Archie being stranded on a sinking ship! Archie, however, has slept better than ever, chalking up his best sleep shift of 9pm to 8am, so it should be sweet dreams all round!

September 13 – 12 Weeks

So, Archie was christened and didn't cry once… even though he was wearing a dress. Everyone agreed (except Tom) that he looked adorable. Even the grey-haired vicar said it was making him broody as he took our little bundle and poured the water over his head.

Nearly 50 friends and family turned out to celebrate with us and it was back to ours after for a barbecue in the garden. Luckily, with all those people to accommodate, we'd been able to borrow some trestle tables and plastic chairs from the little church hall a few doors down from our house. In an array of 70s colours, Tom branded them 'hideous' and tried unsuccessfully to arrange some seat covers at the last minute. I told him we just needed to adjust our mindset.

"They're retro," I said. "A lot of the guests are coming down from London; they'll just think we're really funky."

No one said anything about the chairs anyway, and everyone tucked into the tasty barbecue grub cooked by two of the dads from our NCT group, who were roped in to help.

In other developments, Archie has taken to sticking his tongue out. We were worried we'd taught him a bad habit and looked it up on Google.

According to one website, he is imitating our facial expressions and when he does it without prompting he is actually trying to initiate a game! Archie often likes to play 'tongues' at inappropriate times, like in the queue at the bank or in the car via the rearview mirror. This has led to Tom being laughed at by strangers (at least that's why he thinks they're laughing at him – he does have pretty bad taste in shirts).

We've also been trying to do some daily 'tummy time' play, to help strengthen Archie's neck muscles and give the (now bald) back of his head a break. He's not too keen on it if I just lay him on his play mat. He seems frustrated by not being able to see what's going on, but I read a tip to prop his chest up with a rolled towel and this seems to make him happier.

He's not showing signs of wanting to roll over yet, but I have been impressed by the strength of his legs when I hold him upright and he can even hold and shake a rattle. My mum pointed out that by Christmas he'll be six months, so he should be sitting up and able rip the paper from his presents. He'll also be sat at the table in his highchair and having his own little pureed Christmas dinner!

He almost lost a finger this week, well, he *could* have lost a finger. One of my hairs had wrapped around the top of his left hand middle finger. It was so tightly wound round that it had started to cut off the blood supply. I managed to remove it, but there is still a slight indent, even after three days. Who knew a hair could pose such a risk!

Honestly though, it is downright impossible to keep that boy's hands free of fluff and hairy debris. When he's awake, he keeps his fists so tightly balled that I have to wait until he's asleep and his hands relax to pluck it out. I am now also taking this opportunity to trim his nails. I have tried doing it when he's awake but he jerks his hands around so much I always leave him with lethal pointy bits. We were very alarmed to see he'd scratched a prefect 'x' into his forehead the day before the christening. Was this the mark of the devil? No, said Juliette, one of his godmothers, Archie was just helping the vicar out by marking the spot. We'll go with that story I think...

THREE MONTHS OLD

September 21 – 13 Weeks

For something so small, a baby can create a whole lot of waste. Our bins have been overflowing since Archie arrived; especially as my plan to use washable nappies went down the pan. However, I have been determined to minimise our impact on the environment and have been trialling some biodegradable disposable nappies.

I found a great company online, Beaming Baby, which sells various brands of eco nappies and offers trial packs. I ordered samples of their own brand nappy, plus Moltex (had received good reviews) and Nature Babycare (the only brand available on the high street, at Waitrose and Boots).

I've got to say that I've been impressed with the absorbency of all three. I was expecting some leaks, but I didn't encounter any, even with the Beaming Baby nappy that I tested overnight. Unfortunately, none of them encountered any poo, but Archie's is usually paste-like, rather than runny, so I imagine they'd cope just fine.

One negative is that they were all quite bulky. I selected 'midi' sizes, which fit 9-20lbs (Nature Babycare), 8.5-20lbs (Moltex) and 11-18lbs (Beaming Baby). The Pampers New Baby Size 3, which I have been using, only fit up to 15lbs, so are a bit lower profile.

I also found the nappies a little rougher to the touch, but they all fitted well and smelled nice. Crucially, they did not have the alarming chemical smell, which the Pampers' nappies emit once wet.

Beaming Baby purports to use 30 per cent fewer chemicals than standard nappies, be chlorine free, breathable and 65 per cent biodegradable, including packaging. They state that most of the nappy breaks down within four years, compared with the average 500 years a standard nappy takes.

The other brands make similar environmental claims, but how do they compare on cost? Without buying in bulk, Pampers New Baby size 3 works out around 18 pence a nappy. Looking at similar sized packs, Beaming Baby comes in at 20 pence, Nature Babycare at 19 pence and Moltex – the most expensive – at 33 pence. However, it must be noted that if you were to buy a 136 pack of Pampers, you would only be paying around 8 pence per nappy. Still, this is not really about money, it's about not costing the Earth.

But, having delved a little deeper into the science behind bio-degradation, I'm afraid to say that simply switching to eco nappies might not be enough to save the planet. That's because organic substances only break down quickly when they're exposed to microorganisms and oxygen, and you don't get much of either in landfill. Items of food have been found in a recognisable state after 25 years, so nappies – no matter what they're made from – stand very little chance.

The only other option is to compost them, but considering this process will require an extensive composting unit and still take years, it is sadly just not an option for us in our rented home. So, the conclusion? I have decided to use Nature Babycare, as I can buy them locally and avoid any delivery charges. I may still be packing them off to a big hole in the ground, but they are manufactured in a more ecologically friendly way and they are friendlier to Archie's bottom. Definitely worth the extra pennies.

September 27 – 14 Weeks

A layer of green slime descended on our home this week. We all came down with a cold after a stay with some friends, John and Laura, and their two-year-old twins.

We knew something was wrong because Annabel, the little girl, woke up continuously through the night screaming and by Sunday morning her nose was streaming. Like all toddlers, the concept of germ control, was not something she was familiar with and consequently there was snot being sprayed all over the place. Archie didn't stand a chance. Sure enough, by Monday night he'd started snuffling – as had Tom and I.

I had been dreading Archie getting his first cold. I knew it had to happen sooner or later and that it was *only* a cold, but the thought of him struggling to breath and being unable to help was horrible.

As it turns out, Archie's a trooper and has dealt with it very well, while I have sniffed my way through about 200 tissues and a whole box of Lemsip. There's not a lot you can do for a baby with a cold, but I picked up what I could in Boots, including a saline nose spray and some Calpol. Neither was particularly successful; it was a struggle to get the nozzle of the spray up Archie's little nostrils and when we did, the spray induced tears and screaming, which only exacerbated the mucus fest. Then, when we tried to give him the Calpol, he promptly sicked it back up again.

Laura had told me about Calpol suppositories, available on prescription. So the following day we called the doctors and asked for some. I was a little apprehensive about administering it, but it actually popped up very easily and Archie didn't even seem to notice! He had a nice sleep afterwards and then woke up with a real appetite, so I knew he must be feeling a bit better. This morning, however, he woke at 4am coughing and seemed very distressed, so we decided to make an appointment with the doctor, just to be on the safe side.

By the time we got to the surgery, however, he'd had another bum pill and was actually in pretty good spirits, smiling at the doctor as he examined him with his stethoscope.

The doctor said that bronchial viruses are common in children at this time of year (indeed, the waiting room was full of them coughing away) and not to worry unless he got too wheezy to feed or developed a high temperature.

One cold relief, which I was able to administer easily, was Olbas Oil sprinkled on a muslin cloth. Archie seems to like nothing better than a muzzy - he can spend hours lifting one up and down over his face, peeking out with one eye or waving it about in the air. Forget expensive Fisher Price gadgets with music and flashing lights, we now know just what to get him for Christmas!

Meanwhile, he actually seems to be enjoying his croaky throat, after discovering it can make some fun noises. He's been happily chatting away to himself. If only we knew what he was saying... If I had to guess, I'd say it probably goes something like this: "Can I have some nice new muzzies for Christmas please? I really love playing peek-a-boo with them. Oh, and some milk; I love that too. Thanks Mummy and Daddy; you're the best! By the way, what do you think of my new husky man-voice? Pretty neat, eh?" You see, who needs the Baby Whisperer?!

October 4 – 15 Weeks

Honestly, we've been up and down to that doctor's surgery like a yo-yo recently. Last week it was with Archie's first cold, this week it was for his second set of jabs and then an unexplained bout of crying and fussing during feeding.

He'd start each bottle as usual and then after a few minutes would be howling with pain. He'd be pulling his legs up and arching his back, as if suffering from excruciating wind, but burping him seemed to offer little relief. The agonising screams would go on for about 15-20 minutes and then he'd finish his feed off, as if nothing had happened. We realised that the symptoms had come on about four hours after his jabs, so we called the doctor to see if it could be related. He told us to bring him in for a check, where Archie once again presented the doctor with a big gummy grin, as he prodded and poked (we wondered if he was perhaps putting it on, just so he could see the funny man with the beard and the hugely amusing stethoscope). The doctor gave him a clean bill of health and we apologised for being hypochondriac parents.

"Don't worry," he said. "You'll know you're coming too much when we start giving you loyalty points."

The explanation he gave for Archie's out of character behaviour was raised glands in his stomach – a possible side effect from the vaccinations, which contain small amounts of live viruses. Tom and I both admitted we had no idea there were glands in our stomachs, but apparently, we have glands all over our bodies.

Anyway, something else we both have on our bodies is unwanted fat, and to that end we have employed a personal trainer to give us a few sessions before we sign up at the gym. Kim directed us through a vigorous workout in the living room, while Archie looked on with much fascination and amusement. We even had her weigh us and measure our bellies, which we both had to force ourselves not to suck in!

I was surprised at how stiff and unfit I felt as she led us through squats, triceps dips and one-minute bursts of cardiovascular activity. I was also surprised when I experienced a TENA 'Ooops Moment' while star-jumping, I had thought my pelvic floor had survived the pregnancy unscathed, since I no longer leak when I sneeze (thank god), but clearly I still need to do a bit of tightening up.

Seeing me struggling, Kim was very kind and gave me scaled down versions of the exercises. "It's normal," she said "your body's been through a lot."

And encouragingly, she thinks I can be feeling as fit as a fiddle in as little as six weeks time, if I get active at least three times a week.

Archie, meanwhile, is packing on the pounds without so much as a care in the world. At three months, he weighs nearly 14lbs now – that's a whole stone! No wonder I feel so creaky; it's from hauling around that little lump!

October 11 – 16 Weeks

Before Archie came along, I remember Anna, who has four kids, was forever buying new pushchairs. She'd sell them five minutes later in order to buy a different one, extolling the virtues of the latest model. I used to think she was mad; like an oestrogen-fuelled petrolhead, but just recently I have been hit by the buggy bug. I am totally obsessed. I have spent hours this week checking out online reviews, demos on YouTube and searching for bargains on eBay.

I've been unhappy with my Mothercare Xtreme three-wheel travel system for a while. Equipped with a heavy-duty suspension, it's great for off-roading, but around town its large size is a real pain. It's darn heavy too, making it awkward to lift in and out of the car boot.

I bought it online when it was on offer at half price, without going in store to test drive it first. A novice mum error, indeed. I also didn't appreciate how brilliant the ISOFIX car seat system is. The car seat that came as part of my travel system is not compatible with an ISOFIX base and I very quickly tired of belting it in and out of the car (especially annoying when it's raining and your back gets soaked as you fiddle about).

We ended up buying another car seat, a Maxi-Cosi, after just a few weeks, but I've been soldiering on with the buggy. However, a recent trip to Brighton brought things to a head.

It started when the quick-release wheel quickly released – while I was crossing the road!! A kind lady helped me across and supported the pram (and the perturbed baby within), while I fumbled about trying to fix the wheel back on.

However, the pram seemed to have developed a violent shudder, so I made my way straight to a Mothercare store for their advice. One of their sales people took a look and said a washer had probably come loose internally and that it would need to be sent away to be fixed. The pram would be covered under its two year guarantee, he said, and they'd supply me with a loan pushchair while it was in with them – impressive service, but functioning normally or not, the remainder of the day made me realise the pram had to go.

Brighton's Lanes offer a treasure trove of unique independent stores and quirky cafes, but my hefty pram prevented me from enjoying any of them; getting stuck in every doorway, blocking every aisle and generally causing chaos.

And when I came to get the train home, it was even worse. The thing took up the entire doorway area and I felt terribly embarrassed as rush hour commuters tried to squeeze around us, but I didn't know how to take Archie out, hold my bags *and* fold it up all on my own.

So, I resolved to find the ideal urban stroller; super lightweight, narrow and collapsible with one hand. I narrowed it down to two options from my web research, including a Phil and Teds Smart and a Micralite Super-Lite. After much deliberation, I decided upon the Micralite Super-Lite and nabbed myself one on eBay for £100.

It arrived today and I'm delighted with it. It's incredibly light and agile and it looks great too. You can steer it with one hand and it turns on a sixpence. And because it's got pneumatic rear wheels, I just tilt it back and Archie still gets a smooth ride over our stony, pot hole-filled road.

Micralite says the Super-Lite is suitable from six months, but in my opinion the seat reclines far enough for Archie to sit comfortably at four months – he certainly seems to think so too. What's also great is that you can buy adapters to make it compatible with a Maxi-Cosi car seat, so I'll have to get some of those ordered.

Apologies if you have glazed over, I do realise I am now officially a buggy bore and if you don't want to sit next to me at dinner, I'll understand. At least Anna and I will have plenty to talk about!

October 18 – 17 Weeks

Remember that iconic Nirvana album cover with the baby swimming underwater? Well, Archie's first swimming lesson this week wasn't quite like that, but I'm told he'll get there!

We started off by just familiarising our babies with the water; supporting them under their arms and gently pulling them along, floating them on their backs and lightly wetting their heads. A couple of the babies in our group were not convinced and had to be distracted with toys, but Archie loved it. I had suspected he would, given how much he likes his baths.

He didn't try to kick or splash but he was incredibly relaxed and content and I figure that's a good start. I do wonder if being born in the birth pool has made him more at home in the water?

Our teacher, Nina, said that even at this young age, we could start teaching our babies about water safety. She got us to 'swim' our babies over to the side of the pool and place their hands on the edge and say 'hold on!'.

The lesson didn't last very long, as Nina said the babies find it very tiring, but we finished up with a couple of songs and all seemed to enjoy it. There's more to come however, on our third lesson we will be dunking the babies underwater and by the end of the 10-week course, they should be able to swim a metre or two unaided! What's more, we will even get our very own underwater photographs. I'm only disappointed that Archie won't be able to go naked like the Nirvana baby – the pool operates a very strict two layer nappy policy to prevent any foreign objects escaping.

To be honest, I think my hair poses a greater risk to the cleanliness of the pool right now. It's coming out all over the place. Every day, I scoop alarming handfuls of it up from the floor in front of the mirror where I brush my hair and I'm continually picking it off Tom's clothes and Archie's hands. It doesn't help that Archie likes to use my long blonde tresses as a rope. It's a wonder I'm not bald.

I was aware of the phenomenon of post-partum hair loss, but I thought I'd got away with it. I never expected it to kick in now; four months later. I just hope it won't go on for too long, because by my calculations, I've only got a week and a half before I'll start resembling Yoda, and that's not a good look.

FOUR MONTHS OLD

October 25 – 18 Weeks

As soon as you have your first child people start asking when you'll be popping out more. You're there with this brand new bundle of flesh, still trying to figure out which end is up and someone says "so, do you plan on having more" or "is he the first of many, then?" or "oh you'll have to get a little brother or sister for him."

They mean well, of course, but having a baby is such an assault on the senses, you really need time to work it all out before you go committing to a Brady Bunch-sized brood.

Before having Archie, I was pretty convinced one child would be enough for me, although this decision seemed to outrage anyone I told. "You can't. It's cruel; they'll be so lonely," they said. Or "your child will be a spoilt brat," or "it's so much easier when you have two and they entertain each other."

I heartily disagree with all three of these suppositions. Although I do have three brothers, they're quite a lot older and left home when I was still small, so my upbringing was not unlike that of an only child. But I was never lonely as I got to spend lots of time with friends instead. I've known Elle and Gemma since we were tiny and our parents allowed us to have sleepovers and share holidays, which was wonderful. We always enjoyed our time together and weren't at each other's throats like so many siblings.

The old 'two will entertain each other" may be true, but it doesn't always lead to an easier life for the parents. Whenever I spend time with friends with two young children they are continually having to break up fights, quieten down boisterous play and curtail general mischief making. It's exhausting to even watch.

Here are the other reasons I think 'one is fun':

1) It makes good financial sense. I would like Archie to enjoy many opportunities in life, from horse riding and piano lessons to meals out and foreign holidays, and possibly even private education (should good fortune

smile upon us). Paying out for one child to do these things is expensive enough, double it or treble it and you'd need a lottery win to fund it.

2) Your lifestyle does not need to change beyond recognition. One child is easy to take with you when visiting friends. One child does not mean you have to buy a people carrier. One child can (possibly) entertain themselves quietly, enabling you to get on with work/read the paper/sleep. And when said child starts staying at friends' houses, the parents get to spend quality time together – everyone's a winner.

3) One child will benefit from your undivided love and attention. I want to 'be there' for Archie; to read to him, paint with him, teach him his times tables. I don't want to be that harassed mother that doesn't have time to answer her son's "why? how? what?" questions. I want to help him fulfil his potential.

...And yet. I look at this gorgeous creature and can't help but wonder what a sibling might be like. He brings so much joy to every day and is such a lovely baby, I almost feel we'd be fools not to have any more.

Today he started laughing. Properly laughing (at Tom throwing a sock on his face!) and it was just the most wonderful moment.

I think this is one dilemma which will be an on-going battle between head and heart...

November 1 – 19 Weeks

According to my friend Kate, the four to six month stage is the 'Golden Age of Baby'. A time of smiles and laughter, (mostly) unburdened by teething pains, where you can still turn your back without fear the baby will locate a plug socket to lick.

"It doesn't last long, though!" she said, with an unmistakable note of schadenfreude in her voice.

Well, I'm enjoying it while it lasts. Archie is such a little treasure and we're having so much fun together. This week we started a mother and baby yoga class, which is being run by Nadia; the same lady who taught my antenatal yoga.

I was very curious about how it would work - would we be stretching our babies into the lotus position? Not quite; it's pretty gentle but it does provide some really nice mother-baby contact. We started by sitting cross-legged, with our babies lying in front of us and pitter pattering our fingers up and down their bodies. We moved their legs up and down and side to side, flew them above us like aeroplanes and let them 'drop' from our chests to our knees as we strode around the studio holding them.

Of course, we sang songs (rather badly I might add, as no one seemed to be familiar with the words or the tunes) and ended with the same relaxation exercise I loved so much at the antenatal sessions, which involves lying down, covering oneself with a blanket and visualising a relaxing place... However, it wasn't quite as relaxing as it was before – because I had a baby punching me in the head!

Anyway, we both had fun, and after it was time for even more fun; Halloween fun! Archie's little friend Katrina, from our NCT group, was hosting a spooky party (or at least her mum was anyway) and he got into the 'spirit' of things by dressing as Count Dracula!

Tom and I did exchange guilty glances as we painted his little face white and drew on bushy black brows and a pointy widow's peak, but, hey, what's the point in having a baby if you can't dress him up as the undead? He was in good company; with a little devil, a mummy and a number of pumpkins. We lined them all up on the sofa for the cutest photo opportunity. Tom entitled it 'The little sofa of horrors'!

Later that evening, our next-door neighbours were also throwing a Halloween party and we got to put our baby video monitor to the test... it works!

Mum and Dad got to enjoy a glass of hot Glühwein, while Baby was tucked up safely in bed next door – isn't technology great?! Tom wants to see if the monitor will still work down at the pub, but having seen a photo of Archie's vampire costume, my parents are already to threatening to call NSPCC…

November 8 – 20 Weeks

Yesterday, Tom asked me to have a Skype chat with a friend of his who is pregnant with her first child and considering a home birth. It was interesting for me to reflect on my experiences and it got me thinking about all the things I would tell myself if I could go back to before Archie was born.

Here are my top six:

Be prepared: I thought I had been incredibly organised, with the nursery all laid out, equipment bought and birth plan written, but there were a few vital things I'd overlooked. Namely, a proper test of the birth pool. We did inflate it, which was when the electric pump burnt out, but we didn't try putting any water in it. Had we of done so, we would have realised the tap connector was not fit for purpose and saved a great deal of stress and scalded hands!

As I'd also managed to mislay the water pump, poor Tom had to empty the pool with nothing more than a bucket. Then, when baby had arrived and I needed to give him milk in a bottle, I had no idea how the steriliser worked because I hadn't taken it out of its box. And trying to understand an instruction manual with a baby befuddled head was quite a task!

Make home a haven: As soon as Archie had popped out, my parents arrived round – in fact we had to send them to wait at the pub while the midwife stitched me up!

The following day they were joined by Tom's mum and Rosie, so it was a full house. While it was lovely for everyone to meet Archie and be involved, it was just too much. Ideally, visitors should pop in and then pop off again. Tom spent most of the time running round looking after all the guests, while I had a mini breakdown trying to get to grips with breastfeeding and tend to my birth-battered body without the benefit of any personal space.

Although I felt bad when we asked them to leave, it was the right thing to do. As the door closed, Tom and I breathed a sigh of relief and were finally able to enjoy some quality time alone with our new baby.

Relax: I spent the first eight weeks or so of Archie's life in a state of total paranoia; was baby eating enough, sleeping enough, awake enough... was he even breathing? I was cautious to the point of obsession. Discarding milk that had been unfinished within five minutes, continually replacing dummies for fear they had become unsterilised and changing nappies like it was going out of fashion. Unfortunately, Tom bore the brunt of this anal behaviour and had to tolerate me barking orders at him, as if I knew everything about caring for a baby. Ha! She who had never even changed a nappy before!

I'm pleased to say that things have settled down now, and I have relaxed into motherhood... perhaps even a little too much. Tom had to laugh when I suggested that our neighbours might be able to babysit from next door with the use of the video monitor.

"God, you've changed!" he said.

Trust your judgement: When you have a baby, there's no shortage of people offering you advice – much of it conflicting – and it can be incredibly confusing. Even parenting manuals differ widely in the information offered and 'official' sources can be unhelpful, too. I was bemused by the instructions on the formula packet stating that each bottle must be made up by boiling a kettle and then waiting half an hour for it to cool – I don't know many babies that will be prepared to wait more than five minutes when they're hungry.

I discovered that many mums make up bottles of boiled water in the morning and then just add the formula when they come to feed, and in my experience, other mums are the best source of advice generally.

Don't be too hard on yourself: Breastfeeding can be very difficult. Do not suffer in silence – speak to other mothers, go to breastfeeding support clinics - and if it doesn't work out, then just accept that you tried your best. Your baby will continue to thrive on formula, you won't lose a special bond and you won't be any less of a mother.

Do not be bullied by health professionals or anyone else. Like I said before; trust your judgement – you know what's best for you and your baby.

Purchase wisely: I love a good gadget and having a baby enabled me to indulge that love by purchasing all manner of contraptions. Some of which have proved to be worth every penny and others that are now collecting dust in the back of cupboards. Before splashing the cash, talk to other parents to establish if it's a must-have, a nice to have or just a waste of money and then do your market research to discover the best brands and models.

Investing in a 'travel system' pram which is compatible with an ISOFIX car seat, and installing an ISOFIX base in your car, is something I would advise all new parents to do.

Clothes are another thing you should refrain from buying in great quantity – they're in and out of them before you've even had a chance to remove the labels. Hand-me-downs, eBay or charity shop buys make the most sense and go for styles that are easy on and off – getting things over the head of a wobbly, flailing baby can sometimes require eight hands.

Of course, there are many more things I've learned along the way, but I wouldn't want to share them all – the fun is in the finding out!

November 15 – 21 Weeks

The thought of Archie hurting himself fills me with fear. Would I know what to do? And more to the point, would I be able to do it? Not only am I a total wuss when it comes to blood, when I panic my mind tends to go blank. Not a great combo in a crisis.

I've long worried that I'd be caught in an emergency situation and be unable to help, which is why I volunteered as a first aider many years back when I worked on a local newspaper and was subsequently sent off on a St

John's course. All I can say is, thank god no one had an accident on my watch, because I fainted just watching the video on wounds!

When I found out the NCT was hosting a paediatric first aid course, I thought it would be a good opportunity to brush up my skills. It was taught by two bald burly firemen and focused on CPR and choking. Here's what we learned:

Unconscious baby/child

Dial 999 and put the phone on loudspeaker as you perform the following:

- Lay the baby across your lap, or the child on its back. Tilt the head back and lift up the chin to extend the airway.

- Check for breathing.

- If they are not breathing, place your lips over the baby's nose and mouth (for a child pinch the nose shut) and give two rescue breaths. (Bear in mind that a child's lungs are smaller and only shallow breaths are required – just enough to see the chest rising).

- If the baby/child remains unresponsive, check for a pulse by placing two fingers on the inside of the baby's upper arm, or on the child's carotid artery in their neck.

- If a pulse is present, give one slow breath every three seconds and re-check for signs of life every couple of minutes.

- If the child's heart is not beating you will have to perform CPR: for a baby, place two fingers in the centre of the chest, just below the nipples, and perform 30 chest compressions, gently but at a good rate. Your fingers should push down one third the depth of the chest. For a child, you should use the heel of one hand and push down half the depth of the chest.

- Give two breaths, another 30 compressions, then two breaths.

- Keep this cycle going until medics arrive.

<u>Choking baby/child</u>

Dial 999 and put the phone on loudspeaker as you perform the following:

- If the child is old enough, encourage them to cough hard and vigorously.

- Place the baby/child over your knees (for an older child support them in a forward-leaning position) and give up to five firm back slaps with the heel of one hand in between the shoulder blades.

- If the airway is still blocked, turn the baby over and give up to three chest compressions (the same as in CPR). For a child, stand behind them and place your arms around their abdomen. Clench your fist and place it below the ribcage. Thrust it firmly inwards and upwards up to five times. Pause between each thrust, to see if the blockage has been dislodged.

- If still blocked, give another five back slaps.

- If the baby/child stops breathing and becomes unconscious, carry out CPR as detailed above.

We got to test out the techniques on little baby dummies and I was pleased to find that it's not that hard, if you keep a cool head. Beginning to think about weaning, choking is a major cause for concern for me, but I feel somewhat more confident now.

This may sound crazy, but I am often quietly amazed that I have been able to keep my child alive and unscathed for 21 weeks, not because I'm an irresponsible mother, but because they're just such tiny, delicate little things and risk seems to be everywhere!

In fact we had an incident only this week. Tom managed to lock Archie in the car - along with the car and house keys. He was supposed to be coming to collect me from the train station, and called to tell me what had happened just as my train went into a tunnel and the phone cut off. Very reassuring.

Archie had been crying, and I'd told him he'd have to smash a window, but thankfully he fell asleep after a couple of minutes, giving Tom time to call the RAC. They made it a priority case and were there within 40 minutes. The guy was then able to jimmy the door open just enough to insert a long metal rod and fish out the keys. Archie slept through the whole ordeal, as only he could.

Apparently, children locked in cars happens A LOT. Here's some advice we have since been given; get a copy of the car key cut (it will give access to the vehicle but won't start the engine without the electronic chip) and keep it in a magnetic key holder beneath the wheel arch. Failing that, should you need to break a window, break the windscreen. Because it's not motorised, it's the cheapest to replace and should be covered by your car insurance without excess.

FIVE MONTHS OLD

November 22 – 22 Weeks

Salam alaikum! We are just back from a week in Morocco – Archie's first holiday and it was fab! We opted to stay in a nice hotel on an all-inclusive basis so everything would be taken care of and Tom could have a week off from cooking (I know, I've got it good haven't I?).

I was a bit daunted about packing everything we'd need for baby, getting through the airport and the flight, but we received lots of help along the way.

We were allocated 10kg luggage allowance for Archie, even though we didn't have to pay for his ticket, which was enough to bring nappies, formula and cold-water sterilising bags from home. Luckily I didn't need to worry about food as we haven't started weaning yet (I decided to wait until after the holiday), and his pushchair went on for free.

At airport security, we were ushered through a special 'fast lane' and I was allowed to take through Archie's bottles of boiled water. I just had to taste one to prove it wasn't anything untoward.

I was hoping to get a seat on the plane with a baby bassinet, but apparently these are only usually available on long haul flights, so Archie sat on my lap. It wasn't a problem as it was only a 3.5-hour flight and he slept most of the way.

The couple in front of us said once we'd landed how amazed they were – they'd clocked us getting on and had been expecting a less than peaceful start to their holiday.

This was just the beginning of the praise and attention. Archie amassed a veritable fan club at the hotel, with a constant stream of admirers coming to see him – both guests and staff. We took so many pictures of Archie with random strangers; he's going to wonder who they all were!

A dear old couple called Doris and Cyril took a particular shine to him and kept volunteering to look after him so we could have a drink at the bar or finish our breakfast in peace.

When Tom and I go on holiday usually, we like to lie by the pool and read but we didn't expect to get much time to do that with a five-month-old baby. However, it wasn't as disruptive as we'd feared. We would put Archie in his pram, covered by a UV sun protector net and he'd nap in the shade for a couple of hours while we soaked up the sun.

We even got him a little inflatable boat to support him in the pool. We ended up paying way over the odds for it at 100 dirhams (about £7) in a haggling failure, but it was worth every penny as he absolutely loved it.

We didn't get out and about as much as we usually would have, but the hotel had four restaurants to choose from and a lovely spa, where we took it in turns to enjoy massages.

We did brave a trip to the local souk, where we experienced 'real Moroccan culture', purchasing fake Ray-Bans and three pairs of imitation Converse trainers, which reek of rubber (they're made from car tyres, apparently). Oh, and of course, we got the obligatory photo with a camel.

All in all, Archie seemed to have a great time, apart from suffering a touch of constipation, which I guess was caused by the change in water. Meanwhile, Tom was wrangling with the runs, which meant an inordinate amount of the holiday was spent talking about bowel movements, but at least we didn't run out of conversation!

One of the nicest things about the break was the chance for Tom and I to really focus on our brilliant little boy away from the demands of work and home chores. We noticed small developments, like how he reaches out to touch his reflection in the mirror, has developed a real fascination with his toes and how his noises are starting to sound more and more like 'da-da' (it's ok, I'm cool with that; I know it's a lot easier to say than 'mam-ma).

The only thing I missed about home was the separate bedrooms. When Archie wakes up at 5am and starts chatting away to himself, the wall between the nursery and our room is enough to allow us to continue our slumber but that was not possible with full surround sound – and of course, being on his holidays, Archie had a lot to talk about!

Coming home was a shock to the system – not least because of the autumn weather and having to cook our own dinner; there was a litany of disappointments. First we found our TV digi box had stopped working and lost all our recordings. Then I decided to make a head start on the washing and put a load of Archie's stuff on, but had to pull the plug when the washing machine started making an alarming banging noise and spewing water everywhere. Tom called our landlord to let him know, during which call he informed us of his intensions to sell the house next year. And to top it all off, when I checked my emails, my own tenant has announced he will be moving out just before Christmas.

I feel in need of another holiday already!

November 29 – 23 Weeks

I decided to celebrate Archie's five-month birthday with an introduction to the wonderful world of food. My health visitor told me I could start weaning between four and six months, and although Archie doesn't seem to be desperately hungry (he's still sleeping through – lucky us!) he is now weighing in at a rather hefty 16 lbs 12 ounces and has jumped up to the 50th centile, so I figure he might soon need more to sustain him.

I had been looking forward to the occasion of Archie's 'first taste' for some time. I had pictured the scene: Archie wearing an endearing quizzical look as he samples the new texture and taste. This quickly turns into delight and he eagerly opens his mouth for more.

In reality, it couldn't have played out any differently. I selected mashed banana as the ceremonial foodstuff, as I'd been telling Archie about the delights of 'na-nas' for several weeks, and promising him he could try some soon. I sat him in his highchair, put on his bib and Tom got into position with the iPhone so we could record this momentous happening.

He reacted as if we'd given him a wasp to chew. We tried a tiny bit more. He pushed it out of his mouth with his tongue. I ushered it back in. He started retching. He was sick.

I don't think the footage will make particularly heart-warming viewing when we reminisce in years to come. Still, I'm trying not to get too disheartened as I've read an article on weaning which says it can take up to ten tastes for a baby to accept a new food.

I took to Facebook to consult my mummy friends on the matter and was told that the best food to start with was baby porridge or baby rice – a bland, savoury gruel, which could be mixed with his milk.

Another friend agreed that I'd started with the wrong thing: "Banana is disgusting," she said "It always makes me feel sick!"

Perhaps she was right. Maybe he just wasn't digging the banana? I've now been to the supermarket and stocked up with a range of first foods. I chose an Aptamil porridge, which is the same brand as his formula, and mixed it up nice and runny. I can't say it's had a much better reception, although it at least hasn't triggered any more puking. I'm hoping if I'm consistent and keep offering it every day he'll grow to like it.

My friend Kate told me to look on the bright side: "The longer he's happy with just milk the better," she said. "No need to worry about what he's going to eat if you're out and about, getting the food heated up, finding a high chair. It's much less palaver."

I guess she's right, but I did rather have my heart set on Archie being able to join us for Christmas dinner. But as they say; food is for life, not just for Christmas...

December 6 – 24 Weeks

Archie is still convinced we're trying to poison him. I have persisted with the baby porridge but rather than growing to like it, he's grown to detest it. He starts screaming and crying as soon as I sit him in the high chair and put on his bib.

I tried it myself, and it really wasn't that bad, but in case he just has an aversion to the stuff, I also tried some banana and apple puree – same reaction. I'm starting to worry that this is the beginning of a lifelong negative relationship with food, but at the same time feel I shouldn't just give up.

I consulted the mums from my NCT group, most of whom have babies a month or so older, so are always a good source of wisdom. One of them, Marie, is also a nanny and has 'been there, done that' with a number of her client's children.

She told me that she knew her daughter, Phoebe, was ready for weaning when she nicked some food off her plate one dinner time! (This is the same child who has been doing her business on the toilet since four months old). She went down the baby-led weaning route, where children feed themselves with finger food, and Phoebe is now happy to sit there and gnaw on a pork chop!

"It's great," she told me. "She just eats whatever we're having."

Her advice was to stop trying to force solids on Archie and wait a couple of weeks.

"He's obviously not ready," she said. "Some babies just take longer than others.

"There's no need to worry; babies get everything they need from milk up until around 10 months. Until then, it's just about introducing them to new flavours and textures."

She has invited me to go over to her place in the week to witness a mealtime ("bring waterproofs!" she joked) and has kindly offered to lend me a book about baby-led weaning.

I'm not the only one of our group experiencing food issues; Kerry's baby is intolerant to cow's milk and eggs meaning that she has had to eliminate it from her diet to stop it coming through in her breast milk.

When we went for our NCT mum's Christmas meal there was just one thing on the menu Kerry could eat. She also can't consume caffeine or alcohol – now that's a big sacrifice, but she didn't seem too bitter about it.

"It's great, I've dropped two dress sizes!" she told us.

Archie is making *some* headway in the dinner department; he can now hold his own bottle and seems very pleased about it, too.

In other strange developments, he seems to have discovered how to generate electricity with his feet (I knew the child was a genius).

Let me explain, I had Anna and Elle over for dinner and drinks while Tom was away for the night. Archie woke up crying just after 2am and I brought him into bed with me, so as not to disturb the girls who were sleeping in the room next door.

About 5am, he was awake and really active; thrashing about all over the place. I turned over to see what he was up to and was mighty surprised to see bright sparks of light coming off his feet in the darkness! I had to take a second to work out if I was really awake and try to remember if his sleepsuit was glow in the dark or something. It wasn't; what was happening was that the fleecy fabric had built up so much static from where he was rubbing his feet on the bed sheet that it was actually sparking. It really was an incredible sight.

When I told the girls the next day, they didn't believe me.

"Are you sure it wasn't just a result of that vodka you had before bed?" Anna asked.

I'm certain it wasn't, but I shan't be trying to recreate the situation to prove it – I'm genuinely concerned about the risk of setting the bed on fire!

December 13 – 25 Weeks

This week, our amateur eater Archie was given a demonstration in noshing by his little pal Phoebe. We went over to Maria's to witness a dinnertime in full swing. I was amazed to see Phoebe's plate packed with a chicken thigh, corn on the cob, broccoli and potato skins. Maria simply handed Phoebe a piece of food and she would start tucking in. Having just a few teeth did not seem to hinder her progress; she would grate with her bottom teeth and then suck in the food.

It wasn't as messy as I'd imagined either; her catch-all bib stopped errant morsels from falling on the floor and she could simply pick them back out. Although Maria did warn that if Phoebe held onto a piece of food for too long, she was likely to throw it, and to look out for the telltale hand shaking.

Once Phoebe had had enough, she gave a baby sign for 'all done' and Maria fetched her pudding – a whole apple. Maria just grated off some of the skin with her teeth to give Phoebe a bit of purchase. It was incredible to watch.

To be fair, Phoebe is two months older than Archie, but the communication between Phoebe and her mum was still impressive. Maria advised me to start Archie with some well-steamed broccoli or a finger-sized piece of carrot – anything with a handle on it that can be held and chewed.

"Don't worry if he doesn't seem to actually be eating much of it, just sucking it is enough for them to extract the goodness," she said. "I tried some pork chop after Phoebe had been sucking on it and it tasted disgusting – she'd taken all the nutrients out of it."

Maria said not to start reducing Archie's milk feeds and not to try feeding solids when he was hungry, and would be looking for a 'quick fix'. Baby led weaning is all about letting the child discover food in their own time.

She added that you could quickly progress and basically share mealtimes with your baby, allowing them to have things from your plate - providing what you're having doesn't have lots of added salt or sugar or represent a real choking hazard, like a peanut or whole grape.

I've got to admit that the potential for choking does strike the fear of God into me, but Maria said she had only experienced one incident and a swift clap on the back was enough to rectify the situation.

Baby led weaning is recommended from six months onwards as most babies have lost the tongue-thrust reflex by then, which can cause them to gag. By this stage, their gut has also matured enough to be able to digest all sorts of food so there's no need to stick to bland mush.

Overall, it seems like a better approach to me and I will be starting Archie next week, so watch this space.

SIX MONTHS OLD

December 21 – 26 Weeks

Archie, today is December 21 - the winter solstice. It is also your six-month birthday.

So, what developments do we have to report at this significant juncture? Well, possibly not quite as many as we were expecting, but to be fair, you've still come a long way since those early, scrawny, squinting day.

You are now, according to all who know you, 'a proper little boy'. You have a full head of dark blonde hair, which we are fashioning into a handsome choirboy style, and almond-shaped grey blue eyes. You have your mother's pale skin (I apologise for that) and your father's slightly down-turned mouth (he apologises for that).

Weighing in at a solid 17lbs, we call you our 'hunky, chunky, monkey' and simply love our cuddles with you, despite the strain they are putting on our backs!

You haven't quite mastered rolling or sitting up or eating or popped any teeth through, as I had imagined you might of by six months, but I reckon it's because all your efforts are going into mental agility. You are extremely interested in what Mummy and Daddy are doing on their laptops and phones and like to jab away at the touch screens. You like to watch TV, too. You were engrossed by 'The Graham Norton Show', which I let you watch on the iPad for a whole hour, but I'm not sure I should mention that, as it probably doesn't make me a great parent.

You also love watching 'Strictly Come Dancing', 'River Dance' and the ballet, so we wonder if you might be a dancer once you've figured out how to coordinate your legs. Then again, you are also showing a healthy interest in kicking about your colourful football, so who knows? But you are destined for greatness. That is a certainty.

We are very much looking forward to celebrating our first Christmas together, and Daddy has been determined to make it 'the best Christmas ever', adorning the house with fairy lights and decorations. He's ordered a new Christmas tablecloth, special crackers and family games, has been compiling festive recipes and making batches of chutney to give as gifts. You like to sit in your high chair and watch as he busies around in the kitchen. You don't see Mummy in there very much, but I am glad you will be raised as a 'modern man'.

This week you met Santa. You sat on his knee for a photo and didn't even cry, despite his dodgy looking beard. However, you are still to see the little elf costume we have brought you for Christmas Day, so there may be tears yet!

We're a little sad that you won't be joining us for Christmas dinner, however you have found something you like to eat in honour of the season – Christmas cards. You turned the one sent by the church into a soggy mess, but I guess you were just digesting the Christian message…

December 27 – 27 Weeks

This Christmas brought the most fabulous surprise; we're going to have a new addition to our family….

No, not that. A puppy!

Tom devised such a clever ruse that I simply didn't have a clue. I have been pleading for a miniature dachshund since we first moved in together three years ago, and stepped up the campaign as we approached Christmas. But I know they don't come cheap and Tom said we simply couldn't afford one, so I resigned myself to a new pair of boots instead.

We found the boots in the pre-Christmas sales and they were placed under the tree, along with some pyjamas I had also selected.

"Is there any present I don't know about?' I enquired hopefully.

"Are you kidding?" asked Tom and I felt suitably chastised for being greedy.

Not long after this exchange I got a panicked phone call from a friend asking if I could possibly go and collect an 'antique guitar amp' she had purchased for her dad on eBay for Christmas. The seller lived not too far away from us, while she was in London without a car.

"We were supposed to collect it tomorrow, but the seller is now going away and needs it collected today," she explained.

Of course I could help, I said, and told Tom that I would pop over there and fetch it, while he got the roast chicken ready for our special Christmas meal with Rosie, who we had for the weekend.

"Why don't we all go together? We can find a nice pub and eat out instead, as a treat," he suggested.

And so we all clambered into the car for the 15-mile journey. "It's a bit further than I thought," I grumbled as we trundled up dark country lanes in filthy wet weather.

When we arrived, I asked Tom to nip out of the car and get the amp, but he came back and told me there was something I had to come in and see. So, we all traipsed into the little mid-terrace house.

In the front room was a little sausage dog on a cushion with two hamster-sized pups. I still didn't get it.

Tom pointed: "There's your amp," he said.

I was speechless!

I chose a black and tan little boy and named him Teddy (as I'd always planned). Sadly, we couldn't bring him home with us as he's only three weeks old but we stayed for half an hour, giving him hugs and kisses. We introduced Teddy to Archie, but the puppy was so small and dark, I'm not sure he could really focus on him!

Still, I am certain they will grow to be the best of friends. I'm so thrilled he will have a little pal to love and play with and look forward to teaching him how to respect animals.

It was actually a good job that Teddy didn't come home in time for Christmas, as it was somewhat manic, although very enjoyable. Seven family members descended upon us on Christmas Eve – at the very same time as a nasty cough and cold descended upon Archie. So he wasn't in great 'elf' despite his little green costume, but everyone else donned their festive jumpers and had a merry old time.

Archie received a mountain of presents, although not from us, as we figured we'd save the cash while he's more interested in the wrapping paper!

On Boxing Day, Archie met his cousin Amalie from Thailand (my brother's darling 10-year-old daughter) for the first time. She was completely enamoured with him, despite his streaming nose and hacking cough. Unfortunately the bug had him (or should I say us) up six times that night and we took him to the doctor in the morning.

It breaks our hearts to see him so under the weather but the doctor told us we'd better get used to it – it's not unusual for children to be sick every three weeks once they start nursery, she said. Let's hope the New Year brings more than that to look forward to!

January 3 – 28 Weeks

This is rather embarrassing, but I'm going to tell you anyway, as that is the covenant I have made with you, dear reader. You may remember, around a month after having Archie, I asked Tom to have an inspection of my nether regions and report back on any damage. He reported that it "looked a bit different" but he didn't seem too concerned and it appeared to be functioning as it should, so I left it at that and thought no more about it. I also declined my doctor's offer to give it the once-over at my six-week check, mainly because he's a man and I felt a little awkward.

However, during some more meticulous than usual bikini line shaving I noticed something that looked out of place. On closer inspection, I found it was something that definitely wasn't there before; a fleshy lump hanging down inside.

"Look at this," I said to an alarmed Tom, as I threw my legs akimbo and brandished a hand mirror. "Was this there when I asked you to have a look?"

"Yes – I told you it looked a bit different," he affirmed.

"Different! You didn't tell me there were bits hanging out!!" I cried.

I was mortified and quickly took to Google Images to self-diagnose. It was thoroughly unpleasant viewing and made me so queasy that I actually had to lie down for 10 minutes.

Tom told me to stop overreacting and just book a doctor's appointment. So I did – this time with a female GP. The doctor was very reassuring and told me it was a common side effect of labour. She identified that the lump was the back part my vaginal wall, and not my bladder, as I had feared.

I was worried that, in a cruel twist of fate, I was about to become that woman on the TENA Lady adverts who wets herself by the water cooler, who I have always laughed at so heartily.

Anyway, the doctor says I'm to perform pelvic floor exercises twice a day for six weeks and then return for a check up.

Meanwhile, Archie's been having his own problems of a personal nature. He has been struggling to pass poos, which have been of a very solid consistency and I think he's suffered an anal tear. This is causing him so much pain when he does go that he's started holding on to his poos, making the situation even worse.

Tonight I actually had to help him go. I noticed him struggling, so whipped off his nappy and dived in with a wet wipe. I removed two stone like lumps and was then able to work his legs back and forth to physically push out the rest. It was rather like operating a Mr Whippy machine.

That said, it was significantly less appetising, but it is, I believe, a true testament to a mother's love. Although I doubt it'll be featuring in a greeting card any time soon:

Mum, you've always been there for me,
Given your love endlessly.
You've held my hand and wiped my tears,
Looked after me for all those years.
I want to thank you for all you've done
Even picking the poo from my bum.

What do you reckon?

January 10 – 29 Weeks

It's not easy to get anything done with a baby. Fact.

Overall, Archie is a pretty good kid; he usually sleeps 12 hours a night and can be relied upon to take at least one long nap (of around two hours) during the day – in fact, that's what he's doing right now.

I know that many mums will be green with envy hearing that, but I still find it incredibly hard to get anything meaningful done. Two hours sounds like a long time, but by the time you've booted up the computer, read and replied to a few emails and settled down to work, you're almost halfway through it. Tom blames the Time Bandits.

Try to work when your little one is awake and you spend most of the time nipping back and forth from your seat, alternately feeding, changing nappies, handing over new toys to buy another five minutes, until they decide they are only happy being bounced on your knee and chewing on the computer mouse.

I've been finding it particularly testing recently as I'm trying to get my website finished and establish my little venture, in the hope that I won't have to go back to work come April. I've also been doing some freelance copywriting to bring in some extra income and redecorating my flat while it's in between tenants. Add to that a big dollop of festive entertaining and a sick baby and you've got one very stressed out mummy.

Unfortunately, we don't have any family living locally so I can't ask a granny to lend a hand, as many of my friends with children can. In fact, Tom and I went to a wedding reception last Saturday and we realised it was the first time we'd been out together since Archie was born. Coincidentally, at the baby-weighing clinic this week I bumped into a mum who we'd met at christening preparation. She'd had to go back to full-time work when her daughter was just four and a half months old, and was using a local child minder.

"She's brilliant. She takes the children out and about, does activities with them and is only £4.25 an hour," she told me.

I asked her for the lady's number and gave her a call when I got home. She said she didn't have any space, but put me in touch with another child minder in their group, called Jo.

I only wanted a couple of sessions a week and I was worried that wouldn't be enough but Jo said she was flexible and invited us to visit her. Jo runs her business from home; a spacious bungalow in a leafy lane and only looks after a handful of children at a time. On the day we visited she just had a one-year-old little girl, who was making full use of the mountain of toys on the living room floor.

Jo seemed lovely, as a large folder of glowing testimonials seemed to confirm. And most importantly, Archie seemed really at home there and behaved like such a little angel, it was as if we'd bribed him.

"Is he always this chilled?," asked Jo, cuddling him.

It was tempting to say yes, but we had to admit that he could have his moments.

I really liked the home environment and the fact the children get taken to local groups and out for walks on sunny days. Although we initially thought Archie would attend nursery when he reached 10 months, if he's starting at seven months, this seems like a better option. He is still just a tiny baby and needs the extra attention.... and yes, I do feel guilty about it. However, Jo made the good point that it is much easier to start a child at day care before separation anxiety sets in – usually around 10 months. And at least I have the luxury of starting him slowly.

We agreed on a Tuesday and a Thursday from 10am to 4pm. It is a weight of my mind – finally, I'll be able to get some proper work done... and a good job, too because Archie's just woken up!

January 17 – 30 Weeks

This week has been an extremely productive one. I have written two magazine features, a 1,200 word piece of copy for a client's website, a press release and calculated Tom's end of year expenses. It is amazing what you can get done when you have some uninterrupted time to devote to it.

I did have mixed emotions as we drove away from Jo, the child minder's house, having deposited our most precious possession. However, there's nothing like sifting through a large shoe box of receipts to keep you occupied – yes, that's right, my husband files his business expenses in a shoe box; very professional.

When I arrived later that afternoon to collect Archie, I saw him through the window, sat playing happily. As I entered the room he gave me the most gorgeous big smile and reached his hands out towards me.

Jo said they'd had a great day visiting a soft play centre.

"Archie sat and played with some balls between my legs," she said.

I wanted to say I wasn't sure that was an appropriate activity but held my tongue and stifled a snigger.

She'd started a logbook for him, in which she details their daily activity. Having now started baby led weaning, we'd packed Archie off with a little container of steamed veg batons in the vain hope that he might cooperate and eat it, her being a childcare professional and all that, but the report said: "I was not interested in my veg."

We have now tried broccoli, carrot, sweet potato, pear and banana, which have all been unanimously rejected. He refuses to even pick them up, let alone put them in his mouth. He will have a little suck on a rusk, biscotti biscuit or toast, but still starts gagging if any lumps come off in his mouth, which usually leads to vomiting. I'm afraid to say the thing we've had most success with was an oven chip. He grabbed it off daddy's plate and gave it a good suck.

He has also got a real interest in cups of tea. He gets all excited when he sees us having a cup and tries to grab hold of it (takes after his dad). Obviously caffeine is not great for babies either, but we did put a little bit in a beaker and let him try it. His face lit up when he tasted it, which I think shows some progress, since he's always refused his milk if it's served warm.

Up until now, I hadn't been too worried about Archie's gastronomic disinterest. I figured he's just not ready yet, but other people's concerns have caused me to wonder if I should be doing more.

My parents have been ringing several times a week with new suggestions: Have I tried feeding him a rusk dissolved in milk? Have I tried using a colourful plastic spoon? Perhaps I could try tricking him by putting purée on his teething toys?

I decided to call the health visitor and see what she thought. She advised cutting down his milk from five bottles a day to four so he becomes more interested, but I am reluctant to do this a) because he lost a bit of weight while he was ill recently and b) because my gut feeling is it's not lack of appetite that's the issue.

However, she did say not to worry about it and just keep offering him solids. She said I could try smearing food around his mouth to let him get used to new flavours. And if there was no improvement she could refer him to a food clinic run by a speech therapist.

Having since looked at some mums' forums on the internet, it seems I'm not alone with this problem. But the overall message I'm getting is that babies develop at different paces. He might not be interested in food until he's eight, nine, ten months or more and that's okay, he'll get there eventually. I think they're right. I mean he won't still be feeding from a bottle when he's at university (just drinking from one). I just need to find a way to explain that to other people.

On a positive note, I'm pleased to report things are now improving in the number two department, since the doctor prescribed Archie some special medicine. I took him to the GP because he hadn't had a movement for several days and his stomach seemed to be growing big and round. He had also become incredibly irritable, restless and needy; demanding constant attention (we prayed this was just down to him feeling uncomfortable, and not the first signs of behavioural issues).

The doctor agreed that his anal fissure was probably making him scared to go to the loo. The longer the faeces stays in the intestines, the more moisture is extracted causing it to become hard and thus even more painful to pass – which is exactly what happened to me post-birth so I know just how excruciating it is.

He prescribed dissolvable laxative, Movicol, which he said we could put in milk if Archie wouldn't take it in water. Surprisingly, he didn't seem to taste it in his water at all and we had no problem getting it down him. He had it before bed and by morning a generous package had arrived – a lovely present for Tom!

SEVEN MONTHS OLD

January 24 – 31 Weeks

Ladies and Gentlemen, big news - we have a tooth!

…Not a whole one, but a tooth nonetheless. A sharp little white corner has erupted through Archie's lower gum – proof that he *is* designed to eat solids (although he's still not convinced).

In fact, it has been quite a week for developments. Since we got him a V-shaped pillow and started sitting him up within its safe squidgy confines, he has learned to hold himself up and can even occasionally pull himself back up when he does topple over.

We also treated him to a walker; one that the baby sits in and can scoot about in. It took him a couple of days to get the hang of it but soon he was motoring all over the place. There was such a look of glee on his face as he realised he could finally explore all of the exciting things he'd been eyeing up for so long – like the fridge magnets, the bottles in the wine rack and the dishcloths hanging from the oven handle.

Tom said it was strange having his previously immobile son suddenly tugging at his trouser leg while he cooked dinner!

I'm sure he'll be talking before we know it; he has discovered he can make the most hilarious babbling sound by moving his antique silver rattle (a christening present from his uncle) back and forth in his mouth. We were in stitches as we videoed it and I sent it off to 'You've Been Framed', hoping to snaffle £250. But it obviously wasn't as funny as we thought, as it was rejected.

Another new trick Archie has picked up is shaking his head back and forth as if to say 'no'. However he does it indiscriminately, so I don't think he's using it as a form of communication. I've read that it could be because he's discovered that shaking one's head produces a dizzy sensation, and he's intrigued by it…. just wait until he discovers wine!

The area we would most like to see development in is Archie's movement. He simply will not tolerate tummy time, preferring just to lie like an upturned turtle on his back, making no effort to roll over. A few days ago, I took Archie to see a children's cranial osteopath, as they were offering free sessions at the NCT baby group and I thought it might help.

Cranial osteopathy sounds like a quack medicine. The idea is that the therapist detects disrupted 'cranial rhythms' (whatever they are), which highlight any areas of stress and strain on the body. However, a good friend of mine had taken her son – who was born prematurely and was a very unsettled baby – to see one and swore that he was a different child afterwards.

The osteopath was a very nice lady, who asked me all about Archie's birth. She explained that the birth process is very stressful for babies, regardless of intervention like forceps (although that obviously make matters worse). She came to the conclusion that as Archie spent quite a long time crowning, he suffered additional stress to his neck and shoulders. She spent 20 minutes just feeling him and said she could indeed detect pain in his shoulders. This, she said, was making it uncomfortable for him to lie on his front. So, she did whatever it is she does, and told me I should see an immediate improvement.

And I did. Archie managed a whole 10 minutes of tummy time that afternoon, which is more than ever before. What's more, he was also making froggy, crawling motions.

And this may have been completely coincidental, but he also attacked his rusk biscuit with a real gusto and, I think, even ingested some – fancy that!

So, who knows, maybe there is something in it?

January 31 - 32 Weeks

Archie has a new best friend, and it's black and furry with a wet nose. Teddy, the miniature Dachshund puppy arrived a week ago and the pair are already inseparable.

Teddy doesn't seem to mind Archie pulling his ears, squidging his face or eating his tail one bit, and Archie is quite happy to be clambered all over. We are having to supervise closely, however, as Teddy loves to chew and his teeth, although small, are razor sharp. He doesn't yet understand which are his toys and are ok to munch on, and what's not – such as baby toes, computer cables and our slippers.

Despite the destruction, the way the puppy and the baby interact together really is the most wonderful thing to watch. The minute he sees Archie in the morning, Teddy gets all excited and scrambles up onto his lap, nestling in while Archie drinks his bottle. Archie's little face lights up, too, and he giggles heartily as he watches Teddy maul his favourite monkey toy. What strikes me most is how incredibly similar they are. It almost feels like having two babies at the moment, as I spend the majority of my time wiping up accidents, picking up toys and thrusting chew toys into mouths. The problem is, they seem to prefer each other's teethers and keep swapping whenever I turn my back.

My mother in law was horrified when she saw a video of them playing: "but the dog's licking his fingers!" she cried.

Unfortunately, it's pretty much impossible to keep the situation completely sanitised, but I figure that Archie will be crawling soon and, like most babies, putting absolutely everything he comes across in his mouth… Anyway, being raised by animals never harmed Mowgli, did it?

I've even been taking both babies out in the pushchair, with Teddy curled up in the basket at the bottom. He's certainly stolen the limelight from Archie; people start off cooing over the baby, then notice the super-cute puppy and Archie doesn't get another look in! Tom says he now has the ultimate pulling tools since no woman could possibly resist such an enticing combination.

The cats, on the other hand, are a different matter. Just as they were learning to tolerate Archie, we bring in this little bounding ball of energy to terrorise them. We've had a number of protest pees in the dog's bed and on a beanbag (thankfully made of pleather), which Teddy also likes to sleep on.

On the vet's advice, I have brought in a litter tray for them to use, which does seem to have alleviated the situation somewhat, but just leaves me with more crap to clean up – literally. It's just one long round of pooping and scooping right now, but I can't really complain, seeing as I was the one who wanted all the incontinent creatures. Tom keeps telling me sternly that Teddy "completes our family" and I think I'm inclined to agree.

Away from the chaos of home, Archie and I had a lovely morning at our first Baby Sensory session. It's a baby development class, which utilises lots of different activities to stimulate the babies' senses, including singing, music and signing.

We learned the opening song 'Say Hello' and the accompanying signs for 'sun', 'moon', 'stars' and 'rain'. We played with big sparkly spiders, saw pretty coloured balls bounced around in the dark and discovered a dragon under the sea (an undulating blue sheet with glittery seaweed hanging down, but pretty magical from a baby's perspective).

Now Archie is going to the child minder's twice a week, I'm particularly eager to ensure we spend some proper quality time together and this is just perfect. It's just a shame I can't take the puppy too – I'm sure he'd love it!

February 7 - 33 Weeks

Poor little Archie is *still* suffering from the cough and cold that he caught over Christmas. I keep thinking: "It'll be better tomorrow," but no. We are dealing with one persistent little bugger.

When Tom mentioned it to a friend, she took an ominous intake of breath: "Ooh that's the ten-week cough, that is," she told him.

I thought she was exaggerating, but at seven weeks in, I can see that she was not.

It's not too bad during the day, but every night he wakes himself up hacking away and it's really distressing to hear. I checked the NHS website, which advises to see a GP if your baby has a cough that won't go away. It also warns that a long lasting cough could be a sign of asthma, which is real possibility in our case given my family history (me and my brother have it, and my granddad died having an attack), so we got an appointment to see the doctor.

But, as ever, the GP checked Archie's chest and gave him the all clear. She said that it could be a case of him picking up one bug after another, but added that we couldn't be sure about asthma until he's at least two.

I knew that he'd pick up a lot more germs now he's mixing with other children at the child minder's, but this is ridiculous. He has, however, somehow managed to dodge the chicken pox bullet. I'd been steeling myself for an outbreak ever since we visited Anna four weeks ago and she called the day after to say her twin girls had broken out in spots. The incubation period is up to 21 days, so I'm guessing we're in the clear now?

On the subject of avoiding ailments and injury, we have lowered the height of Archie's cot mattress today. I was unsure when to do it, as it's not like he can pull himself up to standing yet, but he is partaking in some pretty impressive cot gymnastics.

He wriggles about so much, we've had to pad the sides of the cot with folded blankets to stop him getting his limbs stuck in the bars and waking up crying.

What's funny, is that while he sleeps he flips over from his back to his front, turns on his side, wriggles 360 degrees – all of things I try to encourage him to do when's awake, but he resolutely won't. Clearly, he's quite physically capable, but just doesn't want to.

Now he's perfected sitting up and manoeuvring his walker, they are the only two activities he has any time for. I've come to the conclusion that he just won't be a crawler and will go straight to walking.

According to my mum, I was very similar and one day just pulled myself up against the side of the bath and started tottering. Naturally, I will be thrilled if he takes after me. I am particularly hopeful that he will be left handed, like my dad and I, and inherit our creativity (even if that means being as equally rubbish at maths as we are). Us lefties are a very proud breed!

I keep handing him things and seeing which hand he reaches out with, but he refuses to give anything away and just when I think he's favouring one hand over the other, he switches over. Apparently, you can't really tell until they start using a pencil, so he will keep his secret for a while longer. It's just one of many that I'm impatient to discover.

Without wanting to wish away his delightful babyhood, I simply can't wait until he's toddling and talking. I keep having dreams where he's talking to me. Sometimes he just says 'hello Mummy', but other times we have a full on conversation. I'm so excited to hear his thoughts on the world for real!

February 13 - 34 Weeks

Week eight and Archie's hacking cough continues… but hopefully not for much longer. After yet another night punctuated by 20 minute coughing fits, we took the poor little mite back to the doctors and pleaded for help.

This time we got lucky; the doctor *could* hear mucus on his chest and prescribed a course of antibiotics. Obviously, I'm not delighted to be pumping meds into him at fewer than eight months old, but I am pleased we have a course of action that should finally bring him some relief.

I have also been back to the doctors to have a check up on my, ahem, little problem down below. I've been trying to remember to carry out daily pelvic floor exercises but it looks like I need to do more than 'squeeze and release' for a few minutes while watching 'Homes Under The Hammer' because I'm being referred for physiotherapy at the hospital. Even though I can't see any difference from the outside, I must admit that I find the thought of my vaginal collapse quite perturbing. I asked whether it was something that could be fixed with surgery, but the doctor said that was only for serious cases. Apparently it's quite a harsh solution and could lead to very painful sex. In addition, there's simply no point in having it done if there's a chance you might have another child. Even if you do not give birth vaginally the second time around, the weight of the baby can be enough to cause another prolapse. But God knows what happens if you *don't* have surgery to fix it and *then* have another baby – do your innards become your outards?! The thought is certainly good motivation not to find out!

So, anyway, that's all a little bit depressing. On top of that I have a stinking cold, so all in all I've been feeling quite sorry for myself. To make matters worse, our heating isn't working properly and cuts off after an hour, refusing to come back on again until the temperature drops to about 15 degrees. We figure it's a problem with the thermostat but, rather than paying for a qualified heating engineer, our landlord is insisting on fixing it himself. We have to wait for him to come over from France at some point next week, so that'll mean more days huddling by the halogen heater in my coat – no wonder we're all ill.

The winter weather is really starting to grind me down but I am keeping myself buoyed with thoughts of summer. Not only will it bring lighter evenings and warmer weather, but also Archie's first birthday in June – quite a milestone.

Tom and I had said we'd just do something very low key to mark it, but now I'm thinking we should have a BBQ party, invite all Archie's little pals over and get the paddling pool out.

We both have February birthdays, so it's great to have an excuse for a party in the summer months. I'm actually already thinking about his birthday cake – whether he'll actually eat any or not, I have to make him one; it's a mummy's right of passage!

I'm planning a homage to Teddy the puppy; creating a sausage dog body from a chocolate roulade. It's pretty ambitious given my prior cake making experiences (there have been several misshapen monstrosities) but Rosie has promised to help.

Today I got a glimpse at what Archie might be like in five months time, with a visit from one of Tom's friends and her lovely little girl, Frances.

She was ridiculously cute; tottering around the place, putting her arms out for cuddles and passing out toys for us all to play with. She hadn't mastered any intelligible words yet, but it was clear she understood what we were saying to her. It really is the most exciting part of parenthood, witnessing your child develop and become a proper little person.

There's just one draw back to their relentless growth – the ever-increasing weight one's back has to deal with. Holding Frances, I realised I'd have to add another few kilograms to my dumbbells at the gym in order to prepare! Bev, Frances' mum, laughed as I struggled to balance the little girl on my hip.

"She looks so big with you holding her!" she chuckled (I am only 5ft 2in).

Gratefully handing Frances over, I asked Bev how she coped lugging her about.

"I think your body just adapts as your child grows," she told me "I've got impressive upper body strength now".

It's funny that mums are characterised as so soft and feminine, but actually to be a real woman, you've got to be pretty tough!

EIGHT MONTHS OLD

February 21 - 35 Weeks

This week has been a really fun one. Archie is feeling better and it shows. He's been full of beans and at his cheeky, gorgeous, inquisitive best.

Last weekend we bought a playpen and made a lovely den for him full of soft blankets and toys. It had primarily become necessary because of Teddy. While very sweet, he is an extremely enthusiastic playmate and was continually stealing Archie's toys. It was becoming a bit of a stressful situation because there was nowhere in our open plan living space to contain the dog and it meant I was having to closely supervise whenever I put Archie down to play.

However, it's worked out brilliantly because we now have somewhere to chuck all the baby paraphernalia at the end of the day and reclaim the living room for grown up time. And best of all, Archie seems to really like his baby prison… sorry playpen, and I get 20 minutes or so to go about my business knowing he's safely incarcerated.

His new favourite activity is to take objects out of a plastic container shaped like a house. We fill it up with wooden blocks, balls, rattles and chews and he happily sits there removing them all. He gives a squawk when it's empty and we refill it so he can start again.

He's also begun to bang two objects together, which I understand is one of the key developmental markers for babies aged eight to 12 months (cue proud mum moment).

I feel like he's really starting to observe and imitate now. We've had the 'That's Not My Santa' touchy feely book since Christmas and each time I've read it to him I've shown him how to feel the different textures and for the first time this week he reached out to feel them himself, without any prompting (such a proud mummy!).

Encouraged by this and keen to aid his educational advancement, I ordered a set of flashcards. When I received them, I noticed they were for age 18 months plus, but they were only pictures of animals and vehicles and things like that, so I thought he might still like looking at them. I couldn't believe it when I showed him the picture of a cat and he laughed with clear recognition. None of the others seemed to raise any amusement, until we got to the dog and he gave another giggle.

I know how much he loves the animals because he chases them round on his walker, trying to grab hold of them, but seeing his little face light up like that was really surprising (yes, another proud mum moment!).

My good friend Elle, who's a photographer, took some photos of Archie and Teddy this week. It was quite a challenge getting them both to stay still and stop chewing on each other long enough to capture the perfect pose but she managed some stunning shots.

"They look so peaceful and serene," said Tom, looking at them later that evening.

"You have no idea," I laughed. "You should have seen the outtakes. It was more like a baby being attacked by a rabid dog."

"...But it does look like we have the perfect family, doesn't it," said Tom, enjoying his own proud dad moment.

"Yes," I agreed. "But it doesn't just *look* like we have the perfect family; we *do* have the perfect family." I couldn't be prouder!

February 28 - 36 Weeks

To celebrate our birthdays, Tom and I took a trip to Ireland with our little leprechaun. First stop was Holywood, Belfast to visit our friend Lizzie, who herself has a 15-week-old son, Tommy. It was incredibly handy to have all the baby bits on hand, such as travel cot, bouncer, steriliser etc. as we'd bravely travelled with hand luggage only for the long weekend.

Archie seemed to enjoy interacting with Tommy, despite him being somewhat younger and still at that 'do very little besides eat and sleep' stage.

We took a brisk walk with the buggies along the esplanade, admiring the views across Belfast Lough, with its rugged cliffs and beach, and enjoyed lunch in a café attached to a little art gallery. In the evening, Lizzie babysat for us so we could go out to dinner and to the cinema, which was quite a treat. It was actually the second time in a week we'd gone gallivanting (imagine that!), as Juliette, Archie's godmother, babysat last weekend so we could have a slightly belated Valentine's night out.

Lizzie is bringing up Tommy on her own. It was an unexpected pregnancy, but one she was delighted about, as she had spent years struggling to conceive with her ex-husband. He's a delightful little fella (Tommy, that is, not her ex - he's a shit!) and she's managing brilliantly, with lots of support from her mum, but it did make me realise once again how lucky I am to have such a hands-on husband. Our parenting of Archie is split right down the middle and I'm so grateful for that. I'm really not sure I could do it alone.

It was all systems go for Team Mum and Dad when we headed off on the next leg of our journey down to Tullamore (home of Tullamore Dew whiskey) in the south. We'd opted to take the train for the two-hour trip to Dublin and then the bus for an hour and a half to Tullamore, where my oldest friend Gemma lives. It was quite a mission and I think we must have been drinking when we booked it – we certainly wished we had a bottle of the old Tullamore Dew with us for the journey. We ended up in a carriage containing a 20-strong stag do party and sat next to the stereotypical old Irish drunk who insisted in engaging us in incomprehensible conversation for the entire trip.

We then had mere minutes to locate the bus station and meet our connection, which was – naturally – packed to the gills. To make matters worse, Archie had decided that weekend would be a good time to cut three – yes three – teeth, and preventing meltdown required a good deal of distraction. We spent the whole journey passing him back and forth to each other across the aisle, taking it in shifts to entertain him.

Anyway, we made it in one piece and Gemma came to collect us from the bus stop. I knew our stay with her would be quite different to our experience in Belfast. This was a household which would make no concessions for babies and their inevitable noise and disruption. You may remember my account of breaking the news of my pregnancy to her. I knew it was going to be difficult as she's very anti-babies and genuinely thought I was about to ruin my life.

So it was with baited breath that I carried Archie into her house and whispered in his ear to be on best behaviour! He put on an initial good show, playing happily with her two dogs.

"He's nice and quiet," she said approvingly, but still declined to touch him.

The next day, Gemma very kindly treated us to a birthday lunch at the golf club and there was much fussing with high chairs, getting Archie settled and keeping him quiet.

"Eating out's not what it used to be, is it?" she quipped.

I'd been desperate to show her that having a baby hadn't changed our lives, but I guess it has. It's certainly more complicated, but it's also been incredibly enriched. I wanted her to see this, to see his gorgeous smile and hear his infectious laugh, but she never seemed to be looking at the right moment.

Still, I know Gemma enjoyed having us to stay and, once we were home, sent a very sweet text to say the house was very quiet (!) and she was missing us. Give it a few more years and Archie and Auntie Gemma will be the best of friends, I'm sure.

March 7 - 37 Weeks

The most amazing thing happened this week – Archie ate! He allowed me to feed him from a spoon and enthusiastically came back for more. This may not sound like the most exciting thing to most mums of eight-month-old babies, but to me it is a brilliant breakthrough.

It started with a visit to the baby-weighing clinic where I chatted to a health visitor about Archie's exclusively milk-based diet. She affirmed that he was in good shape, weighing a healthy 18lbs 11 ounces, but wanted to refer him to the Dysphagia Eating and Drinking Clinic to have him assessed. She recommended that I try feeding him solids three times a day and asked me to complete a food diary.

The first day we tried baby porridge for breakfast, a finger-food lunch of chicken, green beans and carrot, and vegetable puree for dinner. All was resolutely refused, with the little bugger batting the spoon away and turning his head from side to side and up and down in order to get away from it.

It was the same story on day two, with mush going in every conceivable place apart from Archie's mouth. Come dinnertime, I'd had enough.

"You *are* going to try this," I told him firmly.

I persisted and persisted until I finally got the spoon of creamed baby porridge in his mouth. And guess what? He didn't pull his usual look of disgust. In fact, he seemed to rather like it. The next thing I knew, he was opening his mouth and leaning forward for more. He took hold of the spoon and guided it into his mouth. Then he grabbed the bowl and tried to eat directly from it. He couldn't get enough of it!

I can't explain the elation I felt; my stomach actually flipped! It was just the most wonderful thing to see him finally enjoying something and I rushed to Waitrose to buy two more jars. I was worried that it was just a one-off and that he would refuse the spoon again the following morning, but he did not.

However, we're still taking baby steps; attempting to move on to sweet potato remains a battle of wills. Tom devised a rather mean way of getting it in his mouth; offering Archie his beaker of water and then doing a last-minute switcheroo!

Hopefully we'll identify some more foods that he likes soon – and not all of them sweet and sugary. I mentioned to a fellow mum about Archie's sweet tooth and she asked me what I had cravings for during pregnancy.

"Cake!" I answered.

"Well, then," she said. "Now you know why!".

She has a point, but now he has four sweet teeth I need to look after them. Tom laughed when I came home with a little toothbrush and started poking around in Archie's mouth, but I've got a mouthful of fillings and don't want him to go the same way. I blame my mother for putting Ribena in my bottle. At least Archie loves his water and I shan't be giving him any juices until he's old enough to ask for them.

Although when his baby teeth do fall out, I've seen a great idea on Facebook of how to use it to my advantage – a letter from the Tooth Fairy explaining that she can only make collections from clean and tidy bedrooms!

March 14 - 38 Weeks

Sunday was a very special day; my first Mother's Day (or at least my first with Archie on the outside). I was treated to a lovely lie in, cooked breakfast and a fabulous card with Archie's handprints on the front.

It felt rather strange being on the receiving end of this treatment - not because I'm not used to it (Tom always looks after me) – but because I'm still not used to that label 'mother'.

It sounds so grown up and responsible, of which I am neither. It still feels like the oddest thing to refer to 'my son'. How am I allowed to have a son? I didn't have to take any tests or go to special classes. I just decided I wanted one and hey presto I was pregnant!

Being a parent is such a huge undertaking; you create a human being for whom you must care, nourish, educate and provide for until they are ready to fly the nest, hopefully as stable, well-rounded adults. Sometimes the thought of all that responsibility is overwhelming and I can only hope I'm doing a good enough job.

My niece Amalie came round with her new Furby toy last week. It's a furry purple creature, which wiggles about and makes funny noises – and has no off switch! She explained to me that its native tongue is Furbish, but if you speak to it you can help it learn English. You must also 'feed' it, care for it and love it and its personality will develop. If you don't look after it properly, it might become a 'bad Furby'. It struck me how similar this is to raising a child. Except with a child, it's no game and if you get it wrong, the consequences could be much more serious.

Still, I believe the most important thing a parent can do is love their child, and I love mine very much. I always tell him so, too. Hugs, kisses and praise are also lavishly bestowed. I just hope that makes up for being the kind of mum who leaves her naked baby being entertained by a puppy while she types up a blog, and then turns round to find said puppy licking the baby's winkle… whoops, sorry Archie. I promise not to tell your future girlfriends!

I actually have embarrassing news of my own; I had my first session with the physiotherapist for my sagging innards. She probed me with a white plastic phallus with electrodes on the end and then made me grip it with my pelvic floor muscles for varying amounts of time. I could actually observe the strength of my grip on a computer screen – I'd give a sharp clench and watch the waves peak on a graph, like a seismometer measuring the tremors of an earthquake. This made the whole process a little more fun.

The good news is my down-below strength isn't all that bad, so I won't necessarily become a leaky Laura. The bad news is my prolapse is here to stay, however the therapist has given me an extensive fanny workout routine to tighten everything up. It looks like this will have to replace my actual workout at the gym, which involves kettlebells, as I'm not supposed to lift anything heavy (although that's kind of impossible with a weighty nine-month-old baby). I'm kind of secretly pleased about this, as I now have an excuse not to go to the gym, although I have seen some great toning results from using the weights.

Anyway, I can go back to the therapist again in a couple of months to see what progress I've made. She sent me home with the probe in a plastic bag so we can use it again next time. Except that might be a problem...I could see Teddy out in the garden attacking something earlier – he'd stolen the probe out of my handbag and was having a whale of a time with it. What a dirty dog!

NINE MONTHS OLD

March 21 - 39 Weeks

Archie, you are now nine months old. You have officially spent as long on the outside as you did cooking inside. You have mastered all sorts of exciting new skills since then, which I shall record in this, your fourth quarter report.

This is what the typical day looks like for you: Wake between 7-8am (you now always sleep on your front, which has allowed the little bald patch on the back of your head to fill in), come downstairs, say hello to the puppy and have your morning milk.

Next you will burn off a bit of energy by tearing around in your walker like it's an Olympic sport. You are very adventurous and curious and like to pull all the DVDs off the shelf, chew on the remote controls, pinch our keys and cause general destruction. Sometimes you and Teddy work as a team, with you pulling something out and then dropping it on the floor for him to chew up. Needless to say, this all keeps Mummy very busy.

After breakfast, we go upstairs to get dressed. This is much easier now you can sit up unaided. I love seeing you sat there in nothing but your nappy with your big mop of messy morning hair. It is impossibly cute.

Speaking of your hair, you had your first proper haircut at the barbers this week. Daddy took you and you screamed all the way through! It's much less mullety now, but we still have to use a little bit of mousse to smooth it down. Incidentally, you love watching me blow dry and brush my hair, but you get bored when I'm putting my make up on and make these horrible whiney/growling noises. Another noise you make which none of us like to hear is the grinding of your teeth – you have six now; two little ones at the bottom and two big ones at the top, with two more poking through either side.

If it's a Monday or Wednesday, you'll be off to a baby group for songs and fun or if it's a Tuesday or Thursday, you'll spend the day with Jo the child minder.

You get up to lots of fun things with her – I know because she writes a little report for you every day and keeps a log book of your developments, with photographs.

You like to have a morning nap around two to three hours after waking, lasting around an hour and a half. Then in the afternoon, you will retire again for about the same time. Without wishing to sound rude; I just love it when you're asleep because I can get all my important bits and pieces done, and when you wake up you are always in a jolly mood.

I have been trying really hard to make sure you have three solid meals a day, although this is still a challenge and you may only accept a few mouthfuls. If you decide you don't want any more, you rub your eyes and pretend to be tired, you put your head down to hide your mouth and grab hold of the spoon, to send the food flying. It can be a messy business.

You're not a big fan of our home cooking, but you do like the little Ella's Kitchen pouches of puréed spaghetti bolognaise and fish cakes. However, what you love most are dry snacks, like baby crisps and biscuits. Anything properly nutritious (i.e. fruit or veg sticks) is to be treated with complete distrust.

You are a very lucky boy and have lots of toys to play with. Your favourites change from month to month but right now they seem to be noisy battery operated ones. You are loving the Vtech Discovery Tree, which has little coloured balls to send down a helter skelter slide, and the Playskool ball popper. You get all excited when it springs into life, circling your hands and feet. Today we got you your very own Fisher Price mobile phone, to try and stop you stealing ours all the time (fat chance!).

In terms of motor skills, you are now able to backwards crawl but you get very frustrated that you're not going in the right direction. You can't quite wave yet, but you do make a funny squeezey crab claw movement with your hands. You're good at picking stuff up and can grasp a drumstick to bang a drum, but you're still a little heavy handed when it comes to stacking blocks.

I give you a bath every other day, which you always enjoy, especially as you have now discovered your winkle. You think it's quite a good thing to pull on. I mentioned to my friend that you were going through 'that phase' and she told me it was not a phase, but something that boys and men do for the rest of their lives (sorry if I've embarrassed you).

You love to watch the 'Bedtime Hour' on CBeebies, particularly 'In the Night Garden', which allows you (and me) to unwind before bed. At 7pm, we go upstairs and choose a story. Your favourites are the unseasonal 'That's Not My Santa' and 'Peek a Who?', which ends with a mirrored page in which we can both see ourselves. It always makes you smile.

You are a very good boy and go to bed without any fuss. I put the musical mobile on above your cot and turn on the nightlight and off you go to sleep. I still give you your 'dream feed' at around 10.30pm, which I would like to stop so I can go to bed earlier, but I am afraid of you waking up hungry in the night. Unbroken sleep is such a wonderful thing and I can't thank you enough for that.

They say that around this age separation anxiety kicks in, as the baby realises it is a separate entity from its parents and can be left alone. However, I'm finding it quite the opposite. *I* am realising that *you* are an individual, and not merely part of me. You have your own personality and your own will. It is very strange indeed and a bit scary, but mostly very exciting.

March 31 - 40 Weeks

I wouldn't say I've been dreading returning to work, but I had hoped I wouldn't need to. Unfortunately, it's taking a lot longer than I anticipated to get my new business venture to a point of actually bringing in funds and needs must, as they say.

At the start of my maternity leave, 10 months sounded like such a long time, but it has come round so quickly and I still haven't done most of the things on my 'off work to do list' such as edit our wedding video. Who knew looking after a baby is pretty much a full time job?!

I'm going back to work two days a week, so it's not that painful, but what I do find demotivating is that, after childcare costs, I'll only be bringing home the same paltry amount as the Statutory Maternity Pay I've been getting for doing nothing. Depressing.

Anyway, I had my first day back on Tuesday and it really wasn't that bad. I was surprised to find that I'd forgotten my computer password and how to do a few things inside the content management system of our website, but it all came back to me pretty quickly. And by the end of the day I actually felt like I'd never been away.

In a funny way, working just the two days is enabling me to rediscover what I like about my job. I get to come in, work on a few stories and go home, without the full-time pressure and responsibility.

It's also making me more determined to spend quality time with Archie on the days we do have together. I want to get out of the house, meet up with other mums, go to groups etc.

I was sad that me being back in the office would mean Archie could no longer go to his Wednesday Baby Sensory class, but – for the meantime at least – Tom has decided to take Wednesdays off to look after him. I feel much happier that Archie is only with Jo, the child minder, Tuesdays and Thursdays (my work from home day), rather than three days straight. It had seemed like a bit too much at his young age, but Jo could only offer three consecutive days.

I hadn't felt able to suggest to Tom that he could help with the childcare, he is the main breadwinner after all, but I was delighted when he made the offer.

"Well, what's the point of working for myself if I can't be flexible?" he said.

In fact, he was looking forward to his day of 'daddy day care', he said, although he was a little concerned about being the only dad at Baby Sensory. I assured him that he wouldn't be and that he'd get on just great with the mums anyway. It was true; him being him, he'd come away having learned more about them then I had over the course of seven weeks!

I was impressed that I only got two phone calls from Tom during the day; the first asking directions to Baby Sensory and the second enquiring what he should feed Archie at lunchtime. I was also pleased to receive a lovely picture message showing Archie having fun on the swings at the park and then, come home time, he came to collect me personally.

I could hear Amanda the receptionist coming up the stairs talking in a baby voice and wondered whom she was addressing. Then I saw a little face in the window of the door.

Archie said hello to my colleagues and inspected my desk, so at least he now knows what Mummy's up to when she's not at home. And hopefully he won't grow up thinking Mummy and Daddy spend all day in their dressing gowns doing nothing!

April 7 - 41 Weeks

It's true that you don't appreciate your health until you're sick. This week everyone in our household fell victim to a particularly virulent stomach bug and it was a nightmare situation.

It began on Easter Monday with Archie experiencing a sudden diarrhoea explosion on his play mat, shortly followed by Tom running to the bathroom to chuck up (the latter quite possibly induced by the former!). To give Tom some space, I took Archie and Rosie out to the shops, but by the time we got back, I too had rumblings. Just after 9pm I started vomiting and took to the spare bed, where it continued relentlessly for the next seven hours. At some point during this, I heard more retching from the office downstairs, where Rosie was sleeping. We were dropping like flies.

I was supposed to be going to work and felt rotten having to call in sick, given that I'd only just returned from 10 months off and only work two days a week, but I was too weak to get out of bed. Tom and I thanked our lucky stars that Archie was due at the child minders, since neither of us could cope. Archie hadn't had any further diarrhoea or any vomiting and seemed well in himself so we thought it would be ok. Tom dragged himself into some clothes and dropped him off.

We were just settling down to sip on our rehydration drinks when the phone rang. Archie had filled two nappies within an hour of being with Jo and she understandably couldn't take the risk of infecting the other children. We were beside ourselves. How were we going to care for a sick child (two, actually, as Rosie was still puking) while feeling like death?

There was nothing for it, I decided I would have to call my parents and ask them to come to the rescue. Luckily, they had been visiting friends in Hampshire, so were nearer than normal (they live in Lincolnshire).

They were brilliant; coming to scoop Archie up and whisk him off for a tour of some local garden centres, allowing us to focus on recovering. Of course, we were aware there was a risk of them contracting it too, and we would not have asked unless truly desperate, and sure enough, within hours of them getting back home the next day, it had got them too.

But the bug was not content with six victims, oh no, next we heard that one of our Easter dinner guests had fallen ill and then Jo the child minder, which meant I couldn't go to work again.

The worst thing about it has been Archie's, still on-going, diarrhoea. The continual hosing down, changing of clothes and washing of crap-covered items is truly testing. I've been lucky to have Tom's help holding him down most of the time because otherwise Archie would be putting his hands in it and spreading it across his body and hair. It's horrendous.

It's now Sunday and by the looks of it we are faced with another week of having to keep Archie home and me not being able to go to work. All advice I've received previously is to ensure baby continues to eat and drink and let it run its course, but tomorrow I will be calling the doctor and begging for something to make it stop. Dear God, please make it stop!

April 11 - 42 Weeks

Despite the weekend poo-fest, Monday actually brought a diarrhoea-free day. I breathed a sigh of relief and come Tuesday morning, shipped Archie off to Jo's, allowing me to return to the office and catch up on missed work. All was well with the world.

But just when I thought I'd seen the back of the dreaded runny brown nappies, they made a rampant return. Not long after dropping Archie off yesterday morning, Jo called asking me to come collect him because he'd filled two nappies in an hour and was running a temperature. I left work, feeling guilty for being the 'liability new mum'. However, when I got Archie home, worry took over. I put the thermometer under his arm - 38.8 degrees it read.

I dosed him up with Calpol, put him to bed and called the doctor for an emergency appointment. The doctor said it was possible the gastro intestinal infection had returned and asked me to collect a stool sample just to make sure it was nothing more sinister. She checked him for hernias, chest and ear infections but, thankfully, none of these were the cause.

I asked her if there was anything I could give him to stop the diarrhoea.

"Unfortunately, no. Not when they're this small," she said. "Just keep giving him the Calpol to keep the fever down and ease any discomfort."

Tom's away for work, so I steeled myself for a rough night – but Archie slept soundly and by this morning his temperature had subsided. We actually had a rather lovely day hanging out together. I couldn't get out to my Pilates class, so I did a DVD in the living room, while Archie and the puppy clambered around my exercise mat (which is, in fact, a cot mattress as I'm super professional).

Then I taught Archie how to do a high five, which he found most amusing, and spent the rest of the day sticking his little hand up for me to slap. It was the cutest thing ever.

At lunchtime, I made a little picnic of sandwiches and baby crisps and we sat on the play mat to eat. I held pieces up for Archie to take, but he decided it would be more fun to feed me. He thrust the morsels toward my mouth and was utterly delighted when I took a bite. As a result, I ate a lot more of his lunch than he did, but he was happy.

In the afternoon, we attempted a walk to the park in a break between rain showers, but just as we got to the swings the heavens opened – and I realised that Daddy had inadvertently taken the pram's rain cover with him in the car. We all got soaked – apart from Teddy, who assumed his position in the basket under the pram.

I ran a nice warm bath for Archie when we got back and we settled down to watch a bit of television. 'Mr Bloom's Nursery' is becoming a favourite of mine!

So, it was another day of interrupted work, but I guess there's always time to catch up, whereas these moments with my baby boy will soon be nothing but a memory.

April 19 - 43 Weeks

As much as I love spending time with my son, it's now gone beyond a joke. This is the third week Archie has had to stay at home because of diarrhoea and I've had to cram all my work into his short nap window. The worst part is we still have to pay for the child minder. I understand why, but it certainly adds insult to the injury.

We still don't know what's causing the sickness as the results of the stool test take a while to come back from the hospital. Apparently they have to grow bacteria on the faeces… well, rather them than me.

I'm particularly delighted that this epic bout of the runs has coincided with Archie becoming wrigglier than a maggot. He will not lie still for a second, which makes changing his nappy a four-man job. We have, however, found something to make things a little easier; pull up nappies. I didn't think they made them for babies as young as him and only found out because Tom bought them by accident, but they're brilliant for whipping on and off.

Still, I'm hopeful it's a job I won't have to do quite so many times a day because today has been our first without a dirty nappy in a long time (quite a treat, I can tell you!). Archie also seems much more cheerful and is showing a notably improved interest in his food.

This is a relief because Archie had his 10-month check this morning and the health visitor impressed upon me the need to cut down his milk. He is still having five 210ml bottles per day, which is considerably more than he should be having. I have been trying to reduce it to four, but I'm convinced Archie can count because he protests loudly if we short-change him. The health visitor suggested cutting down the quantity inside the bottle, rather than the number of bottles, which I'm happy to do now he's eating again.

She did point out that by 12 months, most babies should have reduced their milk intake to just two beakers of cow's milk per day. It's hard to imagine we'll be at that point in just two months, but I realise we have to start making more of a concerted effort towards it.

Eating aside, Archie was declared 'a delight' and exactly where he should be in terms of mental and physical development. He weighs 19lbs 5 ounces, measures 2ft 3ins in height, is making the desired 'ba', 'da', 'gah' noises and is showing a keen interest in grabbing hold of things. I was a bit embarrassed that he kept trying to eat the piece of paper towel the health visitor was using to conceal a toy (there's always one 'special' kid who wants to eat the paper, isn't there?), but he totally redeemed himself as we were leaving by giving her a gorgeous wave. I was one happy mummy. And if we have no runny nappies tomorrow, I'll be even happier!

TEN MONTHS OLD

April 25 - 44 Weeks

Someone has stolen my son and swapped him with another baby. He looks very similar, but this one is a complete gannet, eating everything in sight and simply bursting with energy.

We hadn't realised how rotten Archie must have been feeling, but now that he's finally better, he's like a different child. Following examination of his stool sample, the doctor confirmed he'd had rotavirus, a common but vicious bug that nearly every child will be infected with at least once by the age of five.

They routinely vaccinate against it in the US, and apparently have plans to add it to the routine vaccination programme here – unlucky for us that we just missed out.

Although usually not life threatening, it's an incredibly infectious virus that can survive for weeks on hard surfaces like changing tables and toys. And after three weeks of almost constant diarrhoea, it's no wonder that he passed it on to so many others.

Anyway, the important thing is he's better now and he's a joy to be around. The developments in his eating have been phenomenal. He'll eat a massive bowl of porridge or Weetabix for breakfast, an entire Ella's pouch for lunch, followed by a pot of fromage frais and then another pouch for dinner - with plenty of snacking in between! He repeatedly opens his mouth for more like an insatiable baby bird. I can't tell you what a turn around this is; last week I was happy if I could get him to eat a few spoonfuls. I told the doctor about his remarkable transformation in appetite and she said he's probably making up for lost time! If that's the case, it's not just the past few weeks of illness – it's since weaning began.

Now he's finally eating a sizable amount of solids, we have successfully halved the quantity of his two daytime bottles and I intend to halve his dream feed, too.

Jo thinks the effects of Archie's gorging are already starting to show: "His thighs are getting really chubby," she laughed.

Thanks to all the extra fuel, his energy levels have skyrocketed and he's bouncing around all over the place. He's still not mastered the forward crawl but has found a new way of getting where he wants to go by backwards crawling, sitting up and swivelling around. He's trying to pull himself up, too. In fact, he's very focussed on becoming mobile, and while his determination is great, it's also presenting some challenges.

Getting him dressed or changing his nappy, for example, now takes in the region of 20-minutes as he flips over, clambers onto me and grabs hold of anything within arm's reach (my hair, pictures on the wall, every damn sock in the drawer). It's as if life is just too exciting to sit still for even a moment.

Distraction is the key here; I'll get him dressed while he drinks his morning milk or whip off his nappy while he's mesmerised by a musical box. It's really quite tiring, but I'm not complaining. It's so wonderful to see him in good health again, and at least I no longer have to strap him in a straightjacket in order get solid food down him, so we're making some progress!

May 2 - 45 Weeks

A word of advice to the childless, don't make sweeping statements about parenting because you'll most likely have to eat your words when you become one.

I distinctly remember declaring: "I will never be a slave to my baby's routine". The remark came about when my friend Claire, who's son was a year-old at the time, told me that they could not be away from home during the afternoon because of his naptime.

"She needs to relax a bit," a mutual friend and I both agreed. But I finally get it. Upsetting the routine can cause a lot of upset and it's just not worth the aggro.

Tom and I were planning a visit to his mum's, 100 miles away in Hampshire, and decided to set off at 7pm so Archie could go to sleep in the car at his usual bedtime. But, as ever, we found ourselves running late, so we put Archie to bed in his cot for an hour before getting him up again to strap him in his car seat.

Two hours later, we woke him up again to bring him into the house – and this proved to be one disturbance too many. He just would not go back to sleep. He was crying and whinging and nothing I tried to do would settle him. Desperate not to disturb Tom's mum and stepdad sleeping in the other room, I put on the 'Baby Sleep Sounds' album on my iPhone and placed it in the travel cot with Archie. He grasped hold of it eagerly and I knew it would be going into his mouth (in fact, I could hear the volume of the music dipping as it did so) but it was keeping him quiet, so I left it. He finally fell asleep just after midnight and I was able to pry it from his hand. I breathed a huge sigh of relief and attempted to sleep myself, but the respite was short-lived; by 6.20am he was awake again. Seemingly the disruption of his sleep routine had knocked his body clock out of kilter and we struggled with him all day. Come bedtime that evening, he was still having none of it and I spent an hour cajoling him to sleep. It was exhausting and I was cursing being away from home.

As a side note, as a result of his nocturnal chewing, Archie's dribble entered my iPhone's speakers and took several days to dry out, returning them to their full function.

It's not just keeping a routine that I now understand the importance of; there are many other things I thought I would or wouldn't do raising my child which have been turned on their head.

I can see now that I had a very idealised view and the sort of easy smugness that only a first-time expectant mother can have. The truth is, you have no idea what's to come and how you'll deal with it.

I had envisaged some sort of earth mother scenario, where I would carry my child in a papoose while I went about my usual business. The baby would sport fluffy cotton washable nappies, feed from my breast whenever the urge took it and be nourished by the finest home cooked organic food.

In reality, I found myself with a baby who wouldn't suckle, had a messy bout of diarrhoea which gave me a phobia of washable nappies and then refused to eat any solids, forcing me to resort to processed snacks to coax him to eat. Best laid plans and all that.

I'd be lying if I said I didn't feel like a little bit of a failure. I could have tried harder to be the 'perfect' parent, but this is a learning curve for me too and ultimately I have a happy and healthy baby.

I've now done away with parenting books and preconceived ideas. If you ask me, the key to good parenting is just to be fluid and roll with the punches. And if you get knocked down, just be sure to dust yourself off and get back up again.

May 9 - 46 Weeks

We have big news – Archie has mastered a bona fide front crawl! It happened late on Monday afternoon, when we were out on the decking hanging out some washing. Archie was sat at the bottom of the drying rack, pulling his damp socks from the bottom rung (socks are still his favourite plaything – strange boy).

Teddy thought it looked like fun, pinched one and ran off. We shouted at him to drop it, which he did (those puppy training classes are finally starting to pay off!) and the next thing we knew, Archie was on all fours and off to fetch it. To test it wasn't just a fluke, we threw the sock away from him again. He crawled to retrieve it. We did it again and again, cheering encouragement. He looked very pleased with himself indeed and stopped occasionally to wave at the camera I was filming him with (a show off, just like his dad).

This new mobile Archie is taking some getting used to. It was very strange to see a naked baby on all fours suddenly appear in my bedroom, after I had left him on the floor of the nursery wrapped in a towel, whilst I went to fetch something.

"Looks like we'll have to get a stair gate at the top of the stairs," said Tom (we've already got one at the bottom to stop the cats going up).

On top of this notable physical achievement, Archie also pulled himself up to standing in his cot for the first time this week. It's like he feels so strong, having recovered after three weeks of illness, that he's ready to take on the world.

He continues to eat like a piglet and the results are starting to show. In fact, we now affectionately refer to him as 'Lumpage'. I'm not sure exactly what he weighs now, but it's got to the point where I can no longer lift him above my head for 'The Grand Old Duke of York' at Rhyme Time. The waistband on his trousers is decidedly snug and there is a roll of fat under his chin that only a baby could sport and still look cute.

A few weeks back, I expressed concern over whether we would have made the expected transition from milk to solids by Archie's first birthday. I needn't have worried; we have made lightening progress. Since then, I have successfully reduced his milk intake to three bottles a day and last night did away with the 'dream feed' for the first time. I had been gradually dropping the quantity of his final feed over the last fortnight until it was down to just 120mls - and when he didn't even finish that, I knew the time was right to try dispensing with it altogether.

Obviously, we are only one night in, so I don't want to talk too soon, but he slept through without a problem, waking perhaps just fractionally earlier at 7am.

On one hand I will miss that peaceful sleepy feed, where we snuggle in the rocking chair, me deeply inhaling the scent of his baby-clean hair, but on the other, it makes it easier for us all to have an early night. I had also been thinking that soon he would be too heavy to lift in and out of the cot, without waking him.

My friends have started to laugh at the sight of me holding him.

"He's almost as big as you!" they say.

It's true, I am somewhat of a midget and rather slight of build. Rosie is only 13 and already taller than me, which has got to be wrong!

It's hard to believe that Archie will soon be a one-year-old. He seems to be growing up so quickly all of a sudden; crawling and standing and learning new tricks every day.

We will actually be celebrating his first birthday a few weeks early as there is to be a joint party with the other NCT group babies. We have hired the local church hall, organised a secret Santa (or the birthday equivalent) and one of the mums is baking a hugely ambitious cake. I have been put in charge of decorations (my balloon inflating prowess precedes me).

I'm really looking forward to seeing everyone, as we haven't all got together for a while and the babies are changing so rapidly now. I will also be able to properly congratulate Maria - the first among us to announce that she's expecting again! We are all delighted for her, as she was pretty convinced she would not be able to conceive again, following a long battle to get her daughter Phoebe.

There is just one niggling worry about the party; my friend Kate came to visit earlier in the week with her two little boys. Toby, the youngest, was being a bit of a grouch and Kate said he must be teething again. However, later that evening I received a text saying that the real culprit of his bad mood had been discovered – chickenpox.

Archie has already managed to avoid the pox once - will he be so lucky second time around? With an incubation period of up to 21-days, it could see him break out just before the party. I guess we'll just have to watch this space… or should that be spot?

May 16 – 47 Weeks

A couple of years ago, when I visited Beijing in China, I was surprised to see a toddler squatting, with his mother's assistance, to go to the toilet in the middle of Tiananmen Square. I was even more surprised to learn from my guide that this was common practice. Babies in China do not wear nappies and even have specially designed crotchless trousers to enable them to do their business unimpeded.

It's a toilet training method known as 'elimination communication' or EC. It involves the parent closely monitoring the child for signals that it needs to go to the loo, or 'eliminate', and then rushing him or her to a suitable place to do so.

I struggled to see how this would work – it seems hugely impractical - but apparently this method has been used in many countries for thousands of years.

Perhaps it's easier in a country with a warm climate and houses without carpet – a bit like toilet training a puppy – but I imagine it would be very problematic having to whip off a snow suit and several other layers when out and about at wintertime. And I'm sure the looks you'd receive from passersby would be murderous if you allowed your child to go for a poo outside the Post Office.

Needless to say, I wasn't tempted to try EC when Archie was born. Even my (pretty half-hearted) attempt at using washables proved to be too much trouble.

I did have a notion of early potty training, however, since reading an article while I was pregnant about a couple who had apparently potty trained their daughter by the age of six months. She would let them know she needed to go by making the sound 'boo boo' and they would ferry her to the potty.

Having had no experience of babies at this point, this story seemed entirely plausible. It was just a matter of maintaining good communication with your baby… and your progeny being somewhat advanced, which mine naturally would be, right?

The realisation that your child is perfectly average and will develop – stubbornly - in their own sweet time is a little disappointing. By six months, Archie could barely sit up unaided, let alone make an identifiable request to be taken for a 'comfort break'. I quickly realised I'd have to revise my expectations.

However, it turns out waiting until they're ready could be the better option. According to another article I read recently, potty training shouldn't be attempted until the age of three, for fear of causing long-term harm. Author of 'It's No Accident', Dr Steve Hodges says, as well as more toilet accidents, early potty training can lead to constipation, kidney damage and even urinary tract infections because toddlers may hold in their bowel movements longer than they should. It is not until the age of three or four that the bladder is sufficiently developed, he says, and until then children should be able to relive themselves freely i.e. in a nappy.

Anna didn't start toilet training her second son Sean until he was nearly three, which I thought was very late. I was living with her at the time and was always asking her when she was going to start, given that he could walk and talk and seemed to understand almost everything that was said to him.

"He's just not ready yet," she would tell me.

I wondered how she knew unless she tried, but when she finally did, it was a quick and painless process – all done in the space of a week.

To me, this indicated she could have done it earlier, but she said it was worth the wait to avoid going too early and possibly elongating and complicating the process.

Clearly, there are many schools of thought on the topic but according to the NHS most UK parents start potty training between 18 to 24 months, with nine out of 10 children dry during the day by the age of three.

That said, there are two babies in our NCT peer group pushing ahead in the toilet department (if you'll pardon the pun). Maria and her daughter

Phoebe communicate via baby sign language and Maria reckons she always knows what Phoebe is trying to say. She has been dangling Phoebe over the toilet for an early morning poo for months. While I was impressed, I didn't attempt to imitate. Maria is a New Age, spiritual type, into homeopathy. She operates on a completely different plane to me. I am simply not that 'in tune' with my son's rhythms.

However, recently I found out that Katrina, a very down to earth Slovakian, has also been getting her son Jack to do his number two's on the potty. "I'm not going to pretend he tells me when he needs to go," she said.

"I simply put him on the potty after breakfast and leave him until he goes."

She added: "The first time I left him nearly half and hour, but he finally went, and now he goes within five minutes."

This I was even more amazed by – I don't think I could get Archie to sit on the potty for a whole minute, let alone half an hour. He also does not run to such a predictable timetable. He might go around 9am for a few days and then, just when I think I've got it nailed, he'll switch it around to 5pm for the second half of the week. He likes to keep me on my toes, I think.

I have bought a special baby seat, which fits over the toilet seat and have twice tried to whip down his trousers and plonk him on it when I've noticed him beginning to strain, but this hasn't gone down well at all. And trust me, a screaming and flailing nappy-less child mid-poo is not something you want to be in close proximity of.

Archie seems perfectly happy to squeeze one out while sat squarely on the floor, which I imagine is quite a hard thing to do – as evidenced by the resultant pancake-flat poos. Sometimes I try to lay him down to ease its passage but he usually just sits back up again. You always know when one's on the way; he sits there with this disarming 10 yard stare, his face flushing pink and making the occasional grunt. It's a bit awkward to watch really. I don't want to traumatise Archie by forcing him to use the toilet before he's ready, but I do want to show him that there's an easier (and more dignified) way to go. Perhaps I'll pick up a proper potty and see what he thinks?

ELEVEN MONTHS OLD

May 23 - 48 Weeks

Archie, I'm writing to you from approximately 30,000 feet in the sky. I haven't seen you for three days now – the longest I've ever been away from you, but there are only a few hours between us now and I'm very eager to see you.

Over the last few days, I've been looking at photos and videos of you on my phone and – as if seeing them for the first time – have been charmed by you all over again.

"What an adorable, smiley, lovely little baby I have and how very lucky I am," I've thought to myself.

It's not that I don't already know that, but sometimes you need to stand back to get a clear view of what you have.

The day before I left, you learned how to clap. I'd been trying to teach you for ages, but you'd usually just stare at me with mild amusement. Ironically, it wasn't actually me you were imitating the first time you successfully brought your hands together to clap. I was feeding you your dinner and 'Pointless' was on the telly in the background. Every time a round ended and the audience began to clap you would crane your head round to look at the screen and start joining in with the clapping. Who knew you had such an appreciation of general knowledge!

I captured this milestone on video, which provided me with a heartbreakingly cute reminder of what awaited me at home while I was away.

I'm sure you're wondering just where I'd gone – Auntie Elle and I had gone on a long weekend to Majorca in a bid to get a few relaxing days of sunshine.

I'd struck a deal with your father: "How about I go away with Elle for a few days while you look after Archie, and then you can go away with one of your friends while I look after him?"

The idea was that it would afford us a few days of undisturbed sunbathing and reading, which is not really possibly with an active 11-

month-old.

Daddy was a little perturbed by the idea at first, unsure he would be up to three days of 'daddy day care', as he calls it, but I reassured him he'd be just fine and he soon came round to the idea when I agreed that, "yes, I wouldn't mind at all if he went to Ibiza for the weekend."

However, when he came down with man-flu (a mild cold) the day before I left, I did feel rather guilty. I telephoned daily to check on your progress, remind him to brush your teeth etc. and was relieved to hear you'd been a very good boy and you were both getting on great.

I was told you both missed me very much, but I wondered if you were really aware I was gone. It made my heart ache to think it might make no difference to you, but on the other hand, the thought of you being aware of me having gone and wondering why I'd left you was even worse.

My daydream turned dark and I pictured what life would be like for you and your dad if something happened to me and I never returned.

The thought that you could grow up without my love, my cuddles and my kisses to comfort you fills me with horror. I apologise now if I squeeze you a little too tightly when I come to collect you from Jo's this afternoon.

They say that absence makes the heart grow fonder and it's true that taking this little break has certainly made me appreciative of all I have in you and your father. I am very blessed, indeed.

I had left you in search of sunshine, which I unfortunately didn't find – it rained virtually the entire time – but perhaps what I needed to realise is that my sunshine is at home.

May 30 - 49 Weeks

Well, it looks like we've had another lucky escape from the pox– Archie made it to his first, first birthday party (he's having three – well, you're only one once, right?) spot-free. We even managed some sunshine for the day and Archie sported a cute little sailor suit, not that his mood was particularly sunny. He obviously didn't get the memo about it being his special day and all, as he launched into grumpy wailing the minute we arrived at the hall.

To be fair, kicking-off at 3pm, it wasn't particularly well timed – he wasn't the only baby ripe for an afternoon nap and a little overwhelmed by the sudden commotion. Consequently, Archie slept through most of the celebrations in his pushchair, but this did offer one distinct advantage – the chance for Mummy and Daddy to relax, enjoy a drink, gorge on party food and catch up with all of the parents.

We realised we hadn't all been together in one room since our very last antenatal class, more than a year ago. It didn't seem like that much time had passed since we were all sporting baby bumps (well, the women anyway), so it was kind of surreal to see all the little ones up and toddling about.

Archie has become fixated with standing up over the last week; hoisting himself up on any and every ledge with dogged determination. As he can't quite walk yet, once he's ready to change location, he simply lets go and plonks his bottom on the floor. It looks rather painful but he doesn't seem to mind – at least his nappy provides some padding!

He's getting very daring indeed; letting go as if to say "look, Mum, no hands!" and balancing on wobbly legs until it looks like he's going to tumble, then grabbing back on again, just in the nick of time – at least most of the time. Accidents have become a daily occurrence; in fact it's not unusual for him to bang his head at least three times in a morning. I'm worried that people will start to think I'm mistreating him with the amount of bruises he's now sporting. I'm also concerned about the long-term effect all this head banging will have on his mental health.

An ex-boyfriend of mine who turned out to be quite the asshole was apparently once knocked on the head with a golf club and his mother has always claimed this to be the cause!

"He was such a lovely boy, before that," she insisted.

Tom read an article this week about a mother who made her child wear a protective helmet at all times. While we both agreed this is going slightly overboard, I can definitely see the appeal.

I feel like I can't turn my back for a second at the moment without risk of my child sustaining a serious injury. Where I used to be able to leave him lying on his play mat and come back a few minutes later to find him in exactly the same position, I now find him sticking feet first out of the toy box or about to eat a battery from the TV remote control. Even if I just nip to the loo, I'm on tenterhooks waiting to hear the sound of wailing.

I was chatting to a colleague at work about this and she recalled a horrifying incident with her twins when they were little (they're just about to turn 18 now). She had popped upstairs for a few minutes, when she heard the sound of breaking glass. As she ran down the stairs she could hear an ominous 'tink, tink, tink' sound.

"My little boy was toddling towards me with the stem of a glass in one hand and the top of it in the other and was clinking them together," she said. "I rounded the corner to see his sister sat on the kitchen floor, surrounded by broken glass, covered in blood and giggling."

Naturally, she went into hysterics, petrified that her daughter might have swallowed some of the glass, but thankfully the blood was only leaking from a small slice on her fingertip which she had then smeared all over her face.

I recounted this tale to Tom last night as I anxiously searched eBay for protective padding for our fireplace hearth – the next accident waiting to happen. It obviously disturbed him as much as it did me, as this morning I found him trying to install the cupboard clips we bought about six weeks ago.

...On second thoughts, that protective helmet is starting to sound like quite a sensible idea!

June 6 - 50 Weeks

As Archie nears his first birthday, I've been thinking increasingly about what I want for him for the future, or more pertinently, what I don't want for him. This week I was going through some boxes in the loft at my flat (I have another new tenant moving in on the weekend) and came across a scrapbook I'd put together when I was 15. Despite the long list of jobs I had to do, I found myself unable to put it down and sat, leafing through page after cringesome, hilarious, tragic page, whilst pins and needles set in in my legs. It was amazing how memories I had completely forgotten came flooding back as I fingered the plethora of old cinema tickets, train tickets, club flyers, beer bottle tops, letters, drawings and completely random items, like a piece of kitchen towel that, according to the accompanying note, my friend had used when eating a Pop-Tart – yeah, I know, I don't get it either?

It was like stepping into a time machine and taking a trip through my teenage mind. It's not a place I care to revisit too frequently. I get the impression I was pretty obnoxious and spoilt and thought I knew it all. I certainly made a lot of bad decisions (there was a lot of underage drinking, which I'm sure had much to do with it).

I don't want Archie to be like me. I don't want him to make the same mistakes I did. I don't want him to drink so much gin that he's sick for two days and I don't want him to scream at me that 'I've ruined his life', while simultaneously slamming his bedroom door.

I want him to be kind, thoughtful and appreciative, to understand the value of money. I want him to be confident but still humble, to respect himself and others. I want to preserve his innocence, or at least stop him rushing into sex before he's ready.

I told my husband that I hoped Archie would take after him instead, but he laughed: "I was a teenager, too. I was always getting in trouble...and into girl's knickers!"

I don't know if this made me feel better or worse; either it's just an inevitable teenager thing, or Archie is inheriting two sets of degenerate genes.

I fear that it will be even harder to install the qualities I desire Archie to have in this present day and age, where kids seem to be raised via social media and are exposed to anything and everything from such a young age.

It makes me shudder to think what he could accidentally stumble upon while searching for something perfectly innocent like 'cute pussies' (try it and see, or perhaps don't). How do you explain that kind of thing to them?! It's bad enough that our local convenience store has magazines such as 'MILF' and 'GILF' (yes, really) right in the eye line of customers queuing for the post office counter.

I asked Tom if he agreed porn should be completely banned. Initially he said it should just be better controlled, but when I challenged him as to the good reasons for keeping porn weighted against the negative effects of children being exposed to it, he faltered.

"Men survived before access to hard core porn," I told him, and he had to agree that they did.

But seeing as an all-out ban on porn is unlikely to happen any time soon, I guess the only other option is to closely monitor what your child has access to. Anna refuses to let her eldest boy (aged 12) have a mobile phone, despite most of his friends now owning one.

"What does he need it for? He's 12 years old," she said. "I always know where he is and how to get hold of him if I need to."

I've got to admit that I quite like the idea of Archie being able to call me when he's out and about, but it would be enough for him have a non-internet accessible device with just a few 'favourite' numbers available to call and text (in fact, I've just done a web search and there is just such a phone, it's called 1stFone).

There is one other option I've heard about, but it is FAR more draconian. It's an 'invisible' app which you can install secretly on your child's phone (or your partner's, if you think they might be playing away!), which allows you to monitor all their activity – listen in on calls, read texts, see web searches.

You can even remotely turn the phone on to listen in to any background noise and you can use it as a GPS tracking device to pinpoint their exact location on a map!

As much as I want Archie to be a good boy, this is going a bit far even for me. In my experience, the more you assert your authority the more kids will rebel anyway. I guess all you can do is lead by example, make plenty of time to listen to their troubles and cross your fingers they didn't inherit those degenerate genes!

June 13 - 51 Weeks

One week from his first birthday and it appears Archie has mastered his first meaningful word – how very exciting! I'm somewhat disappointed to tell you that it is not 'mummy' but I'm glowing with pride all the same. My little boy is joining the wonderful world of verbal communication!

So, anyway, I guess you want me to get to the point and tell you what it is? Well, it happened like this; yesterday morning Tom made a video call to see Archie, as he'd been working away in London for a couple of days. As soon as I turned the iPhone screen towards Archie he got super excited, reaching out for the screen and saying "dad-da, dad-da!". He even tilted the phone down to look behind it, just in case Daddy had shrunk and was hiding there. It was such a sweet response, Tom and I both felt a little moist-eyed.

"Do you really think he was saying 'daddy?'," Tom asked.

I did, and he gave me further proof later that afternoon. We had just returned from a trip to town to have a lovely photograph of Archie playfully grabbing Daddy's sunglasses printed out. I placed the photo in a silver frame to create a little gift ahead of Father's Day this Sunday. Once I'd finished, I turned it towards Archie and said 'what do you think?' Archie smiled and again said "dad-da, dad-da!"

And when Tom went into Archie's room this morning he was greeted with an enthusiastic "dad-da!", so even he believes it now. I really love the relationship they have. Archie's hero worship is clear to see; all Daddy has to do is pull a funny face or pretend to bash into something and Archie is in fits of laughter (he loves a bit of slap stick). I have to work a lot harder to elicit a hearty belly laugh, although I did get one this week, by slapping a book closed at the end of his bedtime story. The more violently I did it, the more he laughed (yes, a little worrying, I know).

I know he loves me; if he hurts himself it's me he wants to have a cuddle with, but for fun-time it's Daddy all the way. Men generally seem to hold a lot more interest for him than women. I think he will be a man's man. My friend Claire said her little boy Liam, who's three, is just the same.

"He's always telling me Daddy is his best friend and that he doesn't like playing with girls," she said. "Even at the supermarket checkout he wants to go to a male cashier."

Anyway, I don't think it will be too long until Archie has a name for me. When I came down the stairs this morning, he saw me through the glass in the living room door, pointed and tried to say something, but nothing really came out. I think we just need to do a bit of work on it; a few intensive 'mam, mam, mam' sessions.

Still, I think it's lovely that his first word of 'dad-da' has arrived just a few days before Father's Day. What a fantastic present for Daddy. It's a good job too, since the original present I had been planning went disastrously wrong.

A word of advice: don't attempt to make plaster cast feet with a 12-month-old. I got the idea from reading a fellow mum's blog. It seemed fairly straightforward and I thought it was a beautiful keepsake idea, so I ordered a casting pack from eBay, complete with gold paint to gild the little plaster feet with once finished.

First you have to mix up the alginate so it turns from white powder to pink slop. The timing is very critical; you must decant the liquid and start the mould before it turns white.

Attempt one, and the pot I'd chosen proved to be too shallow. I couldn't get Archie's foot at the right angle to properly submerge and before I knew it, there was gloop everywhere; all over his hands, clothes, the high chair and the floor. I'm desperately trying to clear it up before any of it goes in his mouth when Teddy runs in and tries to start eating it. Cue profanities.

Attempt two, I try to take the mould in a plastic bag, but all the liquid is spilling out as I pour it in and Archie is not happy at all about having his foot thrust into a load of cold gloop for the second time. He's crying, wriggling and flailing while I try to hold the bag still for three minutes while the alginate sets – three minutes, yeah right. It didn't take me long to realise this was never going to happen.

I considered waiting until he was asleep, but I was pretty sure dipping his foot in a bowl of goo would be enough to wake him. In the end, I cleared up all the mess, stashed the plaster and paint in the cupboard and resolved to wait a couple of years.

So, Daddy's getting a framed photo instead. And, as we know, a picture speaks a thousand words, but he's already got the most important one.

ARCHIE'S FIRST BIRTHDAY

On June 21 - Midsummer's Day - Archie turned one. And before we'd had a chance to give him any presents, he gave me one; he said "mum-mum"!

As it was only last week he learned "da-da", I wasn't expecting this development so soon, but there he was, standing in his cot, grinning and calling me Mum!

Honestly, my stomach flipped. It's hard to describe how it made me feel being identified by him for the first time. It is a truly amazing moment. As new mothers, I think from the moment our babies are born we're looking for affirmation; that we're doing ok, that they're happy, that they're developing as they should be.

I found it quite tough during the initial few weeks, spending virtually every moment catering to the needs of this little thing, which gave *absolutely nothing* back. But when that first smile came at six weeks it all became easier. 'Hey, what do you know? My son likes me!'

Then you start to see a personality emerging from your squidgy blob of flesh, learn that he has likes and dislikes.

In the last month he's become seriously attached to a baby blue bunny comforter, which Granny bought for him when he was born. It's been hanging around in his cot for ages, but it's only now that he's started showing interest in it. He likes to suck its ears; suck them until they are sopping wet. The thing now smells like ditch water and is properly gross. But this is the way Archie likes it. Nay, loves it. He ensures it is returned to this state almost as soon as it's been washed.

He was dragging it around everywhere but we've had to establish an in-cot only rule to give it at least some daily respite. Tom has already been making online enquiries to see if we can source a back up bunny, God forbid this one gets lost.

As grim as the cuddly toy is, I'm kind of thrilled at this demonstration of self-expression and I love seeing how excited he gets when he sees Bunny at bedtime. And to be fair, many would say it's not as bad as my childhood comforter – a dead stuffed fox. I fell in love with it at a junk shop when I was six and my dad bought it for me. I spent the next couple of years dragging it around with me, using its claw to stroke my nose as I sucked my thumb. I finally had to give it up when the paws fell off and the stuffing started coming out (not to mention the fact that I was starting middle school).

It seems like Archie gets more and more 'human' by the day now. If I ask him for a cuddle, he'll come and give me one – well, most of the time. He's independent and likes to help himself to his water beaker throughout the day and to brush his own teeth. He has favourite books, which sometimes he will sit and look at with absolute fascination for about 20 minutes.

He's so close to walking now. I'd thought he might have been able to do it just in time to perfectly wrap up his first year, but I know it's not far off.

He can manage four unsupported steps from Mummy to Daddy before his Bambi like legs give up on him. We were helping him practise yesterday when Tom looked at me and said: "I don't want him to grow up."

I knew exactly what he meant. While every milestone is wonderful, they all seem to be happening so quickly now. I mean there was virtually nothing for months, and then 'dad-da', 'mum-mum' and first steps all in one week! It's like he's reached a tipping point, and next thing he'll be driving and bringing girls home.

I always thought it was such a cliché to say 'they grow up so fast'; a sentiment invented for cheesy TV commercials, but I now understand that they do.

Baby boy is fast becoming a toddler and to celebrate this passing of time we held a big family birthday party at home on Saturday. It was supposed to be an even bigger affair, with 40+ guests invited for a barbeque in the garden but we awoke on the day to dismal rain and gusty winds, which were causing the marquee we'd erected the day before to lilt in alarming directions, so we had to cull the numbers. Even with family members only, there were 16 of us, which still felt like a proper party. Tom cooked the food on the barbeque outside and we ate it inside in the British tradition.

There was birthday cake for afters – yes, I did attempt my ambitious sausage dog design! It was highly complex, consisting of two Swiss rolls for the body, a large muffin for the head, a Cadbury Mini Roll for the snout and fairy cakes cut in half for the legs/feet.

My friend Cathy helped me make it the day before and unfortunately we were both equally clueless when it came to cake decorating. We mixed up some icing sugar and added black food colouring and then slopped it all over the cake construction. We then created big floppy ears, a doggy nose and a long tail from rollout icing dyed black. It looked atrocious. More like a deformed crocodile than a dog but it was too late to go back to the shop.

After Cathy left and the icing had dried, I attempted to embellish the rather sorry looking creation (or as Elle would say, I tried to 'shine a shit'). I added chocolate buttons for eyes and claws, ribbon as a collar and added some 'tan' markings with chocolate squeeze-out icing. I scraped away all the excess icing, which had pooled around the dog's body, surrounded him with strawberries and piped out 'Archie' in icing. It actually didn't look too bad! It was never going to win any prizes but I was happy that I'd managed to fulfil my motherly duty by presenting a homemade first birthday cake (even if I didn't bake it myself).

All the guests managed to suppress their laughter and we got the obligatory photo of child crying as everybody stood round to sing him happy birthday.

Archie got so many presents. We now have an obscene amount of multi-coloured plastic monstrosities that have taken up residence in our living room.

I worry that this profusion of toys is laying the foundations for one very spoilt child, who thinks it's completely normal to receive gift, after gift, after gift (in my day you were lucky to get a single clementine, don't you know!!!).

It's true that he's currently more interested in ripping off the wrapping paper (and eating his cards), but it still feels a bit wrong for him to have so much when there are so many children with so little in the world.

At least Tom and I didn't go mad with the presents. Anna was having a clear out of baby bits, now her girls are nearly four, so we bought a baby 'laptop' and a Fisher Price piggy bank for Archie, both of which he loves... although he still has a lot of time for the pasta-filled milk carton Daddy made for him. Long may he continue to delight in such simple pleasures and delight us daily with his antics.

These past 12 months have been the most eventful, most challenging and most wonderful of my entire life. I have learned so much about myself; I think I may even have become a 'better' person – less selfish, more patient and with more love in my heart than I ever thought possible.

I want to thank my son for the many gifts he's given me, and thank you for sharing the journey with me.

The End

ABOUT THE AUTHOR

Mindy Miller is an award-winning freelance journalist and writer. She has written for national newspapers and magazines, leading online publications and television. She lives in West Sussex with her husband, son and sausage dog.

15316439R00077

Printed in Great Britain
by Amazon